THE

PRIMARY CARE–MARKET SHARE

CONNECTION

HOW HOSPITALS ACHIEVE
COMPETITIVE ADVANTAGE

THE

PRIMARY CARE–MARKET SHARE

CONNECTION

HOW HOSPITALS ACHIEVE
COMPETITIVE ADVANTAGE

Marc D. Halley

ACHE Management Series

Health Administration Press

Library of Congress Cataloging-in-Publication Data

Halley, Marc D., 1955
  The primary care–market share connection: how hospitals achieve competitive advantage/Marc Halley.
     p. cm.
  Includes bibliographical references.
  ISBN-13: 978-1-56793-275-1 (alk. paper)
  ISBN-10: 1-56793-275-4 (alk. paper)
  1. Hospitals—Economic aspects. 2. Medical care—Marketing.   I. Title

  RA971.3.H22 2007
  362.11068'8—dc22

                                                            2006046997

The paper used in this publication meets the minimum requirements of American National Standard for Information Sciences—Permanence of Paper for Printed Library Materials, ANSI Z39.48-1984. ∞™

Acquisitions editor: Janet Davis; Project manager: Jane Calayag;
Layout editor: Chris Underdown; Cover designer: Trisha Lartz

Health Administration Press
A division of the Foundation of the
   American College of Healthcare Executives
1 North Franklin Street, Suite 1700
Chicago, IL 60606-3529
(312) 424-2800

Contents

Acknowledgments

The material for this book is a culmination of years of consulting and management experience with many people in a variety of circumstances too numerous to list individually but critical to acknowledge collectively. First, I acknowledge those with whom I have journeyed. Their hard work and insights, often in the face of significant challenges, have contributed to my understanding and to our organizational intelligence. Second, this work would not have been possible without the strategic laboratories provided by numerous clients in several states over several years. While my team and I entered each consulting and management engagement armed with correct principles, we left with new learning and best practices that magnified our experience. Special thanks to those clients whose leaders had the courage to implement change. Third, I must acknowledge special mentors who shared their counsel and support, particularly my father, who encouraged me to write.

My personal thanks to those who have been with me during our launch of The Halley Consulting Group, LLC, including William Reiser, Michael Ferry, Brian Morton, Robin Walters, Ashleigh Knill, Michelle Wier, Andrew Halley, Regina Elkins, Karen Bridges, Kerri Brown, and last but not least, Lisa Reiser. These are the implementers of correct principles, the purveyors of best practices, and the substance behind the theory.

To Debbie and our brood

—Marc D. Halley

Introduction

Some of the ideas and perspectives presented in this book, particularly ideas about market share and competitive strategy, run contrary to the prevailing view of the hospital as the center of the healthcare marketing universe. As I emphasize throughout the book, if the success of a business is based on capturing and retaining market share, hospitals and invasive specialty physicians[1] are poorly positioned to do so.

Traditional measures of market share, which revolve around hospital admissions and discharges, are merely measures of throughput. While invasive specialties put huge dollars on the hospital revenue line, they do so on the basis of cases (again, throughput) rather than market share. Both hospitals and specialists are critical to healthcare in the communities they serve, yet both are highly dependent on referrals and are therefore potentially vulnerable to an astute competitor who understands that primary care providers attract, retain, and direct most patients or customers. The true measure of market share is the number of primary care providers (each of whom retains somewhere between 2,000 and 5,000 patients in a practice) who prefer a hospital and its affiliated specialty physicians and will refer patients to both, as the occasion requires. In short, ***primary care = market share***, and the success and affiliation of primary care providers should be the concern of hospital strategists, group practice executives, and specialty physicians alike.

The concept of primary care providers (both physicians and others) as the holders of market share dramatically affects my view of sustainable competitive advantage. Despite the trend toward developing more sophisticated service lines, despite brand identity, despite community image, and despite the trend toward employing specialty physicians, referrals from primary care physicians drive the success of most specialty practices and most hospitals. (Yes, I know all about emergency department volumes and the resulting admissions, but those numbers will not be enough to sustain most acute care facilities.) Very few "Mayos" and "Cleveland Clinics" exist in the United States that can claim even regional name recognition. Most providers operate in an environment where achieving true sustainable differentiation in the minds of consumers in a single community is difficult at best. Consequently, a sustainable competitive advantage must begin with a primary care strategy—what I call "retail strategy"—that is integrated with specialists, service lines, and hospitals. The resulting continuum of services captures and retains patients and their money (or insurance) in the system before competitors can do the same. (Just owning a few—or several—primary care practices does not qualify as a retail strategy.)

At this point, some readers may think that the concepts in this book are just more of the same "integration stuff" we tried and failed to achieve in the 1980s and 1990s. My career has spanned both decades, and I am firmly convinced that nothing was wrong with the integration model. We (myself included) fouled up the implementation because we treated everything as a department of the hospital rather than as a unique business with different rules for success. We are seeing this same blunder committed by some hospital executives today, as they build or acquire primary care and specialty practices and employ physicians.

Hospital and health system executives who are looking to increase or protect direct referrals from primary care providers, or indirect referrals from primary care providers through affiliated specialists, will find the concepts presented in this book essential to their success. Based on my consulting experience in multiple markets, both large and small,

I am convinced that those who stick with the standard "build it and they will come" mentality and who ignore the need to attract primary care market share will ultimately succumb to more astute competitors. Sole community hospitals are also at risk from limited-services providers (e.g., ambulatory surgery centers, diagnostic imaging centers), some of which operate below the radar, even in certificate-of-need states. My colleagues and I have occasionally been called on to work with hospitals that are attempting to catch up with competitors that have already captured market share in their numerous affiliated primary care practices. The challenge of coming from behind, especially in markets with slower population growth, is almost overwhelming—politically, strategically, and financially.

This book presents a different perspective on the concept of integrated medical services. Here, I offer a competitive model based on the needs, wants, and priorities of various customers (including referring physicians) and the roles of physicians and hospitals in meeting those needs, wants, and priorities to achieve a sustainable competitive advantage. Hospital executives, whether they are managing single service lines or entire regional systems, will clearly understand the importance of placing affiliated primary care providers throughout their primary and secondary markets to capture and retain market share—one small community or neighborhood at a time. They will also clearly see the critical role of relationship management in connecting their affiliated specialists to this captured market share and in attracting referrals to the hospital and its various services. Readers will understand the vital role of the hospital chief executive officer in managing what has been termed a "demand chain" (Blackwell 1997).

This book is for those who provide medical services rather than products or financing. I apologize to readers who are seeking a discussion about the critical interrelationships among services, products, and payers. My decision to focus largely on service providers is not intended to discount those relationships or the essential role of each component of this complex industry we call healthcare. Instead, this book is an attempt to clarify, to simplify, and to focus on a particular aspect of properly integrated medical services.

Hospitals and health systems continue to focus the majority of their capital dollars on bricks and mortar, new equipment, new service lines, patient satisfaction programs, and now the employment of specialty physicians. All this investment, some of which is absolutely necessary, presumes that patients will come if we have the facilities, equipment, and services available and if we promote them effectively. What this presumption ignores is the reality that as consumers we do not worry much about those services (most of which we cannot even pronounce) until we need them. Then, unprepared to make decisions about complex medical issues, most of us are totally dependent on our "regular doctor" to guide us through the maze of healthcare alternatives and risks. That regular doctor is likely to be a primary care provider whose preferences and affiliations will dominate his or her referral decisions. I contend that hospital executives and strategists should spend as much energy and capital on capturing their market share in primary care practices (owned or affiliated) as they do on preparing to meet complex clinical needs. Rather than concentrating on the back end of the food chain, we must look at the front or opposite end, where "Mrs. Smith" makes the majority of healthcare purchasing decisions for her family and where primary care providers deliver the majority of the services she selects.

NOTE

1. For our purposes, invasive specialties include all the surgical specialties and others whose practices are procedure oriented (e.g., invasive cardiologists). Patients generally do not self-refer to invasive specialists. Noninvasive specialties include those who provide largely cognitive services.

REFERENCE

Blackwell, R. D. 1997. *From Mind to Market—Reinventing the Retail Supply Chain.* New York: HarperCollins.

The New Competitive Model

This chapter[1] presents three concepts:

- Traditional hospital strategies
- Medical group evolution
- The new competitive model

CONCEPT 1: TRADITIONAL HOSPITAL STRATEGIES

In most markets the competitive healthcare-delivery battle traditionally has been fought hospital to hospital. A number of competitive strategies have been used over the past few decades, and the majority of these fall into one of the following categories:

- Traditional workshop strategies
- Service-line strategies
- Practice ownership
- Medical staff development

Workshop Strategies

Years ago, new hospital administrators would make their presence known in a community by remodeling the hospital entrance. Those were the days when workshop strategies were king. Bricks and mortar were the dominant competitive factor, and investment capital for facilities and equipment was the primary driver during budget discussions. "Average age of plant" was considered a critical measure of competitive potential. Common workshop strategies include the following:

- A great geographic location within a reasonable distance from growing suburbs
- A constantly updated physical plant
- A number of convenient and accessible operating rooms
- New labor-and-delivery rooms
- Capital for physician-requested equipment
- Convenient transcription services
- Convenient physician parking
- An attached medical office building
- Breakfast in the doctor's lounge
- A fine nursing and clerical staff
- One or more physician liaisons promoting services and soliciting feedback
- A physician referral service
- Ask-A-Nurse® to assist with primary on-call issues
- Relationship-management activities on the part of the chief executive officer (CEO) and senior managers
- Continuous process improvement
- Convenient access to lab and radiology results

The problem with workshop strategies is that they are difficult to sustain as a competitive advantage. For example, the impact of one new construction project might last just long enough for the competitor to complete its new building or remodeling project. Under the certificate-of-need (CON) laws that existed in many states, some workshop strategies had the potential to result in a sustainable competitive advantage. However, as CON laws have been modified or replaced and as well-heeled competitors have moved into many markets, the competitive advantage of workshop strategies that revolve around capital projects has proven unsustainable. In recent years, with advances in technology and nonhospital sources of capital, physician groups have created their own workshop strategies for many of the most profitable diagnostic and therapeutic procedures traditionally performed in the hospital, and they have implemented those strategies even within CON states.

Workshop strategies involving human resources have traditionally been no more sustainable than strategies based on bricks and mortar. Competing facilities generally have drawn from the same pool of employees within the community (particularly for professional staff). Hiring practices have not routinely focused on recruiting the professionals whom Bradford Smart (1999) calls "A-players"—the top 10 percent of available talent for a particular job at a particular wage or salary. Similarly, hospital managers (some of them "C-players" themselves) have not been willing or able to redeploy their poor performers. Instead, most healthcare organizations have harbored a number of C-players. Consequently, competing hospitals have shared the same bell-curved profile of managerial, professional, and clerical staff.

In most markets workshop strategies are still relevant, but they have become the minimum ante required to remain in the competitive game. A reasonable average age of plant, access to capital, efficient and well-managed operating suites, a fine nursing staff, and convenient parking are required just to play. A hospital located in a high-growth, high-income suburb has some potential advantages over a central city facility, but even these advantages can be and frequently are overcome by less well-positioned competitors. In short, workshop strategies are rarely a source of sustainable competitive advantage.

Service-Line Strategies

In the 1980s and 1990s, as workshop strategies proved less sustainable, hospitals adopted a service-line or "centers of excellence" approach to achieving competitive advantage. Service lines proved to be quite a bit more sustainable in most markets, with emerging heart programs leading the way. Many service lines required not only new facilities and technology but also the acquisition and development of specialty teams and unique processes that were more difficult for competitors, even those with adequate capital reserves, to duplicate. The sustainability of some service lines was (and in some states still is) facilitated by CON laws, which protected hospitals from free-market competition. Early on, competitors in many communities seemed to operate under a silent pact, with one facility developing a heart program, another becoming the cancer center, and so on. Most developed some expertise in labor and delivery, first building labor-and-delivery rooms and then labor-delivery-recovery-postpartum suites. Before long, however, the gloves came off and competitors began pursuing each other's market share in profitable programs.

In most competitive non-CON metropolitan markets today, multiple programs exist in heart care, cancer treatment, orthopedics, and other profitable service lines. In some large metropolitan markets there may be a dozen or more heart programs, including programs owned by for-profit investors and physicians, that are all competing for patients' attention. Sustainable differentiation in such markets is difficult if not impossible. Rather than being a source of sustainable competitive advantage, possessing one or more successful service lines is the minimum ante in many markets today.

Practice Ownership

In the late 1980s many hospitals began acquiring primary care practices and employing primary care physicians as a defense against the anticipated onslaught of managed care. These primary care providers (PCPs) were to offer hospitals critical access to "covered lives," which would be controlled by managed care plans. As gatekeepers, PCPs were to control (or restrict) access to specialists and hospitals under a capitation approach. This approach was expected to reduce the medical-loss ratio for payers and maintain risk pools for providers. However, the predicted flood of managed care and capitation did not materialize in most markets. Worse, most hospital investment in primary care practices was a disaster. In fact, hospitals actually reported $80,000 or more in annual operating losses per employed physician (HealthCare Advisory Board 1999).

By the late 1990s the cry of divestiture was heard throughout the U.S. healthcare system, and some hospitals successfully divested their practices without apparent consequence. In more competitive markets, however, many of those who pruned or eliminated their investment in primary care practices noted a corresponding loss of market share. Former employed physicians left the community, shifted hospital and specialist affiliation, or became employed by competing hospitals. This phenomenon should not have come as a surprise, but it did.

The gatekeeper strategy seems to have been doomed from the beginning. However, the primary care strategy still has tremendous competitive potential if it is focused on capturing and retaining market share and if properly implemented. When hospitals acquired primary care practices in the past, their focus was on developing a lever for use in negotiating with managed care plans and maintaining access to capitation risk pools. Successfully entering the primary care business with the intent of capturing and retaining market share was only rarely the prime directive. Hospital-owned practices traditionally have been money-losing ventures, primarily because the decision makers lacked an understanding of the rules for success in the primary care business. Also contributing to the demise have been a limited vision and understanding of the practices' strategic value in capturing and retaining market share for the hospital and affiliated specialists and a narrow grasp of the multiplier effect of a dollar spent in a primary care office.

Medical Staff Development

Another common competitive strategy was the recruitment of physicians to the hospital workshop medical staff. Traditional medical staff development efforts focused on building and maintaining service lines and recruiting enough primary care physicians to quell the demand for more PCPs from specialists, who are dependent on primary care referrals. In most cases, these efforts yielded little more than a recruitment list supported by community need data. Although the term "integration" became popular during the 1990s, very few hospitals consistently focused attention on connecting their specialists with PCPs and on connecting both to the hospital. Instead, the traditional "build it and they will come" mentality dominated most strategic plans. Hospital CEOs and senior managers focused their attention on invasive specialists who placed direct revenues on the hospital's income statement rather than on PCPs, who actually created groups of customers and kept them.

CONCEPT 2: MEDICAL GROUP EVOLUTION

Medical Practice Consolidation and Expansion

Medical practices did not fare much better at achieving competitive dominance. As reimbursement declined, as the business of medical practice became more complex, and as quality of life became a priority for younger physicians, groups began forming at a tremendous rate. Solo practice, particularly among the non-invasive specialties, was no longer acceptable to most physicians completing residency programs. Group practices—with their employment options, the perception of having less financial risk, and offer of better quality of practice and on-call life—became the norm in communities of all sizes. Single-specialty groups formed in many specialties, and multispecialty groups expanded as practice consolidation occurred. Physicians circled the wagons to pool their resources and protect themselves. Some groups focused on achieving a competitive advantage by opening satellite offices or rotating through distant primary care offices or small community hospitals. Others recognized the importance of PCPs as sources of referrals to specialists and began hiring and placing these physicians in convenient geographic locations. Still others reached the size and acquired the capital needed to purchase more invasive diagnostic and therapeutic technology within the large group-practice setting.

Physician Practice Management Companies

In the 1990s, with the development of publicly traded physician practice management companies (PPMCs), huge amounts of capital became available to large group practices to fund their competitive strategies (and also promised wealth through stock options). Many large practices succumbed to this financial temptation and entered into lengthy management agreements. Part of the allure of PPMCs was the promise of independence from hospital capital and workshop dominance. Also alluring were the ability to access new technologies and the revenue-enhancing opportunities that were previously available only to hospitals and health systems.

By the late 1990s the PPMCs, once the "darlings of Wall Street," had lost their sizzle (Hochman 1998). The house of cards collapsed, and with the collapse hundreds of millions of dollars in stock value melted away like hoarfrost on a sunny morning. The promise of capital and professional management was gone, replaced by lawsuits, embarrassment, and debt for many fine multispecialty and some single-specialty groups. As for sustainable competitive advantage, group size and location yielded an advantage for some groups in some communities, but not to the exclusion of competitors who wanted to enter local markets.

CONCEPT 3: THE NEW COMPETITIVE MODEL

Hospital and health system executives, large medical group leaders, for-profit chains, and other healthcare organizations are still struggling to find a sustainable competitive model that will maintain or enhance their share of the healthcare market and the financial returns associated with competitive dominance. A new model that is emerging in some markets is built on a foundation of workshop and service-line strategies. Yet the true source of sustainable competitive advantage lies in understanding, developing, and effectively maintaining what I will call "retail" and "demand chain" strategies (Blackwell 1997, 2). The development of a truly sustainable competitive advantage lies not in the hospital, the surgery center, or the multispecialty medical group. It starts with the customer—the end user of the services.

Peter Drucker (2001, 164) stated that the prime directive of a business enterprise is to "create and keep a customer." Neither hospitals nor invasive specialists (who put most of the revenues on the hospital ledger) actually capture or retain the end user of medical services. Instead, they have cases or admissions that last a relatively short period of time. These service providers are identified as "occurrence providers." Primary care providers and some noninvasive specialists, on the other hand, are considered "relationship providers" (Halley 2002). Figure 1 lists some of the medical services provided in each category.

While occurrence providers clearly have "customers," they do not usually maintain relationships with these end users. Conversely, relationship providers have the opportunity to build long-term associations with patients at the end-user level. As the most common access point for medical services, relationship providers both attract and retain these customers. In fact, the true measure of market share and market potential for hospitals and specialty physicians lies not in admissions, discharges, or procedures, which simply involve throughput, but in the number of primary care practices affiliated with these occurrence providers. Some PCPs initially are offended by the term, but they are, by definition, the healthcare equivalent of "retailers." The power that these physicians potentially wield, and rarely use, is significant.

According to Louis Boone and David Kurtz (1977, 289), "retailing consists of all the activities involved in the sale of products and services to the ultimate consumer for his or her own use." For most end

Figure 1. Medical Services of Occurrence Providers and Relationship Providers

Occurrence	Relationship
• Hospital inpatient	• Family medicine
• Hospital outpatient	• General internal medicine
• Emergency departments	• Pediatrics
• Surgical specialties	• Obstetrics
• Rehabilitation and therapies	• Internal medicine subspecialties
• Ancillary services	• Long-term care

users, PCPs are the point of sale or access to the healthcare delivery system. When our fictional customer Mrs. Smith (who makes the majority of the healthcare decisions for her family [Braus 1997]) moves to town, she does not select a hospital or a general surgeon in case she or a family member requires these services. Unless there is a preexisting condition within her family, Mrs. Smith will not seek out an otorhinolaryngologist, a perinatologist, or a pathologist. Instead, she will choose from among four or five primary care specialties those physicians through whom she and her family will access healthcare services. She will likely select a family practitioner, a general internist or pediatrician, and an obstetrician. Her selection of PCPs will then directly affect her use of more invasive specialty services and her choice of hospital, if and when these services are needed.

Many PCPs maintain almost total control over the selection of specialists for their patients. Patients are sent to the PCP's specialist of choice and, by default, to the hospital or system affiliated with that specialist. Because of the trusting relationship that PCPs have built with their customers, they can refer the majority of patients across town, against natural retail-migration patterns, and past other hospitals and specialty physicians to the specialist they (the PCPs) prefer. These PCPs also have a significant ability to directly admit patients to their (the PCPs') hospital of choice. Thus, building a retail strategy around a strong primary

Figure 2. Traditional Product Supply Chain

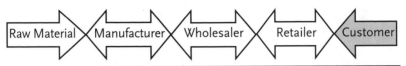

care base is increasingly essential for hospitals and invasive specialists in competitive markets.

Hospitals and single-specialty and multispecialty groups that understand the principles of retail strategy will increase their market share by affiliating with adequate numbers of PCPs, each of whom may capture and retain 2,000 to 5,000 patients (or "covered lives," to use the managed care term). The competitive challenge then becomes how to legally and ethically capture the referrals from affiliated PCPs. This is the realm of demand-chain management.

Figure 2 illustrates the standard retail product supply chain (reading from left to right) for goods produced and delivered through retail outlets. The process starts with consumer demand (reading from right to left) for products, which is met at the retail store by retailers who have, in theory, anticipated that demand and ordered the products from wholesalers, who ordered them from manufacturers, who in turn made them with raw materials ordered from other vendors. Similarly, Figure 3 illustrates a simple medical services supply chain (reading from left to right), showing the delivery of services, from the most invasive diagnostic and therapeutic procedures performed in hospital settings to the least invasive cognitive medical services provided in primary care offices. The demand process usually starts with a patient (Mrs. Smith) who goes to the doctor (most often a PCP). Based on the patient's need, the PCP may send the patient to a specialist or directly to a hospital for more invasive procedures, including hospital-based physician services. Both the retail product supply chain and the medical services supply chain highlight the fact that demand for products and services is triggered by links close to the ultimate customer.

Figure 3. Medical Services Supply Chain

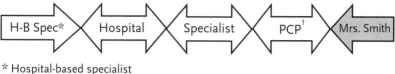

* Hospital-based specialist
† Primary care provider

In his book *From Mind to Market: Reinventing the Retail Supply Chain*, Roger D. Blackwell (1997, 2) says that successful organizations will increasingly focus on consumer-driven demand chains, which integrate all the components of the supply chain around a singular focus—meeting the expectations (demands) of the retail customer, the "ultimate master."

The interdependence of medical services providers creates a natural demand chain with some unusual characteristics. Figure 4 illustrates the unique "customer plurality" associated with the medical services demand chain (reading from right to left). Unlike participants in the supply chains for most industries, where only the retailers see the end user, each member of the medical services chain interacts directly with the "retail" customer. In addition, each succeeding step along the chain must meet the unique needs, wants, and priorities of every chain member in all of the preceding steps.

This phenomenon presents both a tremendous challenge and an opportunity for participants in the medical services demand chain. The challenge lies in ensuring that each demand-chain member clearly understands and is prepared to meet the needs, wants, and priorities of the retail customer and of all the preceding demand-chain members. The opportunity lies in the interdependent nature of the medical services demand chain, which requires that all members of the chain work together to ensure a positive overall experience for the retail customer. In fact, failure by any member of the demand chain contributes to a negative customer experience and therefore reflects poorly on all other demand-chain members. For

Figure 4. Customer Plurality of the Medical Services Demand Chain

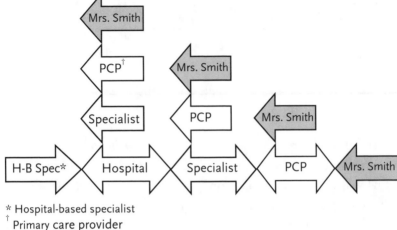

* Hospital-based specialist
† Primary care provider

example, an accurate preliminary diagnosis that is confirmed by a technically superior invasive diagnostic procedure, leading to a flawless surgical procedure, which is then unfortunately followed by inferior postoperative nursing care, results in a negative experience for everyone involved. This places all demand-chain members (not to mention the patient) at risk.

In an era of consumerism, those organizations that learn to unify demand-chain members around meeting the needs, wants, and priorities of the customer (the retail customer as well as other demand-chain members) will have a sustainable competitive advantage.

MANAGING THE DEMAND CHAIN

Blackwell (1997, 1–2) emphasizes the importance of managing an entire demand chain to ensure a successful customer experience:

> In the new millennium, the rule of battle will be rewritten. No retailer, manufacturer, or wholesaler will be strong enough to win on its own.

Great firms will fight the war for dominance in the marketplace not against individual competitors in their field but fortified by alliances with wholesalers, manufacturers and suppliers all along the supply chain. In essence, competitive dominance will be achieved by an entire supply chain, with battles fought supply chain versus supply chain.

Some of the most successful retailers and manufacturers of the past two decades have achieved their competitive advantage by effectively integrating some or all of the components of their supply chains and focusing those elements on meeting the needs, wants, and priorities of the retail customer. Some of these successful integrators have elected to own all or portions of their chains. Others have taken a leadership role in managing or influencing the entire chain to achieve retail customer focus.

The strategic implications of effectively managing the medical services demand chain are significant. Healthcare providers are painfully aware of the challenges associated with integrating demand-chain components. Unfortunately, many integrated delivery strategies focused on responding to "the managed care threat" or a competitor's attempts at integration, rather than on meeting the needs, wants, and priorities of retail customers. The failures of the prior two decades prompted the late-1990s' trend toward "dis-integration" and divestiture.

THE BOTTOM LINE

Given the current consumer-choice environment, it stands to reason that the most successful and sustainable competitive strategy will be an integrated medical services demand chain built around a solid primary care retail approach that focuses on understanding and meeting the needs, wants, and priorities of the retail customer and other demand-chain members and that does so better than competing delivery chains. Ownership of the demand-chain components will be far less important than the ability to unite efforts and ensure consistent, high-quality care and caring. Those who succeed will capture and retain the retail customer and the flow of referrals that are so critical to the success of affiliated specialists and the affiliated hospital.

The sustainability of this new competitive model lies in capturing and retaining the retail customer in primary care practices and in legally attracting referrals from these practices to other demand-chain members rather than losing them to competing demand chains.

In reading this chapter, some hospital executives and physicians will immediately write off the new competitive approach as just another integrated delivery model. They will discount the potential of successfully working together when they appear to be competing for an adequate slice of a seemingly shrinking revenue pie. Meanwhile, their wiser competitors will be going about the business of capturing and retaining market share in outstanding affiliated primary care practices and attracting that market share into superior specialty and hospital services focused on meeting the needs, wants, and priorities of retail customers and demand-chain members. The resulting market-share shift will likely be permanent.

NOTE

1. Some sections of this chapter were originally presented in M. Halley. 2004. "The Case for a Medical Practice Retail Strategy." *The Journal of Medical Practice Management* (November/December): 163–66. Used with permission from Greenbranch Publishing, Phoenix, MD.

REFERENCES

Blackwell, R. D. 1997. *From Mind to Market—Reinventing the Retail Supply Chain.* New York: HarperCollins.

Boone, L. E., and L. D. Kurtz. 1977. *Contemporary Marketing, 2nd ed.* Hinsdale, IL: Dryden Press.

Braus, P. 1997. *Marketing Health Care to Women.* Ithaca, NY: American Demographics Books.

Drucker, P. F. 2001. *The Essential Drucker.* New York: HarperCollins.

Halley, M. D. 2002. "The Case for Divestiture." *Carolina Healthcare Business* (July/August): 19.

HealthCare Advisory Board. 1999. "Stopping the Bleed: Reversing Losses in Owned Practices." Washington, DC: The Advisory Board.

Hochman, R. L. 1998. "PPMC Accounting Practices Draw Scrutiny." [Online article; retrieved 11/07/06.] http://library.findlaw.com/1998/Oct/1/131280.html.

Smart, B. D. 1999. *Topgrading: How Leading Companies Win by Hiring, Coaching and Keeping the Best People.* New York: Prentice Hall Press.

CHAPTER 2

The Retail Customer

This chapter presents four concepts:

- The customer as the center of the universe
- Retail customer behavior
- The risks of purchasing healthcare services
- Making your market

In most medical practices the center of the universe is the physician. The practice offers the services the physician is willing and able to provide, on the days and at the times the physician prefers and according to the physician's preferred style of providing those services. That style reflects the physician's training, personality, life stage, gender, and, even, hobbies. The smaller the medical practice or department (in a multispecialty practice), the more pronounced the personal influence of the physician or physicians on service-delivery options.

The center of the universe in the hospital setting is a bit tougher to single out. Likely candidates include invasive specialists,[1] who place a great deal of revenue on the books; powerful and profitable service lines; bricks and mortar; and, of course, the expense side of the income statement, which becomes the clear winner during lean financial times.

But should these people and items be the center of the universe in the healthcare setting? Let's consider another possibility—the customer.

CONCEPT 1: THE CUSTOMER AS THE CENTER OF THE UNIVERSE

Most hospitals and many medical practices go to great lengths (and expense) to measure patient satisfaction. Some use very sophisticated tools to monitor their patients' satisfaction with the individual components of the services provided. Practices want to know how well their receptionists, appointment desk staff, and nursing staff function. They want feedback on the patient's impressions of the physician and whether the patient would refer friends. Similarly, hospital executives want to know about the courtesy and efficiency of their admitting staff, the helpfulness of their nurses and technicians, and the perceived quality of their meals. Many of these organizations use the results of their surveys to identify and correct shortfalls in customer service. They often are quite successful at improving their scores and therefore their service. Still, most medical practices and hospitals do not seem to be interested in making the customer the center of their universe. Why not?

We have heard much about the "consumer choice" environment and its effect on those who provide products and services of all types. Russell Coile (2002) described the implications of this new environment for healthcare:

> In a consumer-choice environment, patients have the option to select almost any hospital and physician. Providers can "make their market" by out-competing rivals in offering best-in-breed technology, physician specialists, service, and facilities.

While Coile's conclusion was certainly critical, it illustrated the classic "if we build it, they will come" workshop strategies that have dominated our traditional approach to doing business. Let me offer a modification to Coile's conclusion that places the end user—the "retail" customer—at the center of our universe: In a consumer-choice environment, patients have the option to select almost any hospital and physician. In the absence of any preexisting condition, they will do so by first selecting a primary care physician or PCP, usually one recommended by a friend or relative who has had a positive experience with that physician. Hospitals and specialty physicians can "make their market" by successfully implementing strategies that will attract business from PCPs who control the majority of referrals to specialists and to hospitals.

A high-tech image, a broad range of specialists, great service, and fine facilities are indeed critical to success in most markets today. However, the keys to developing and sustaining a competitive advantage are capturing and retaining the retail customer in affiliated primary care practices and organizing the entire demand chain to meet not only the customers' clinical needs but also their non-clinical needs, wants, and priorities and doing so better than competing organizations.

These nonclinical needs, wants, and priorities are important. Consider that healthcare providers are highly trained and intent on meeting the clinical *needs* of patients. Medical training, equipment, and facilities are, of necessity, focused on meeting those clinical needs. Unfortunately, most patients have a difficult time recognizing clinical quality and competence, even if quality and competence are the characteristics that distinguish one medical services demand chain from its competitors. Providing great clinical care is essential, but it is not enough.

In the consumer-choice environment, healthcare providers are called on to meet the demands of patients who behave more like customers than patients. Gone are the days of patients patiently waiting to see a physician. Gone are the days of blind compliance with the counsel of a trusted medical adviser. Physicians today are faced with customers who have "wants" and "priorities," such as convenient appointments, an interactive discussion of their condition or the latest wonder drug they saw advertised, and a second opinion if they do not get the answer they want to hear. Hospital-based physicians, nurses, therapists, and others experience the same challenges when they try to meet the expectations of patients and their families—expectations that may have little to do with the patient's clinical care.

Every provider in the medical services demand chain personally interacts with retail customers, so let's look at these customers' purchasing behavior. This way, we are better prepared to identify and more appropriately meet their needs, wants, and priorities.

CONCEPT 2: RETAIL CUSTOMER BEHAVIOR[2]

Customer behavior is influenced by the nature of retail service delivery. The perceived risk associated with purchasing services (including healthcare services) is higher than the perceived risk associated with purchasing products. Consider, for instance, the purchase of an automobile. A tremendous amount of comparative information about almost any vehicle one might consider acquiring is readily available to the consumer. With relatively little effort, one can gather data on performance, reliability, quality, individual features, routine maintenance costs, price, financing, resale value, and so forth. Armed with this information, the potential buyer can test-drive and compare alternatives. The buyer can solicit opinions from her social circle about their general experience with automobiles and about the particular style under her consideration. In short, a plethora of purchasing information can be obtained with little effort. A vehicle purchasing decision presents some risk, but the availability of information and the ability to touch and test-drive the product minimize that risk, allowing the buyer to develop a reasonable impression of the value associated with the vehicle and then helping her determine whether to make the purchase. Smart product retailers often provide money-back guarantees to reduce any remaining risk perceived by the buyer.

Except for recognizing the simplest of medical procedures, most patients usually cannot even spell much of what they experience in a physician's office or hospital. The kind of information commonly associated with product purchases is not available for medical procedures, and patients often have a difficult time assessing the clinical value of various medical options, even if the procedure or treatment and its risks and potential outcomes are clearly explained. They often are totally dependent on the medical professional who will provide the service personally or will refer them to a specialist. PCPs sometimes give their patients the opportunity to choose a specialist, but they admit that the majority of the time the patients are referred to the physician's preferred specialist. It is unlikely that the patient comes to the primary care appointment having already researched and selected a few cardiologists, for example, just in case a referral is necessary. The patient depends on his trusted PCP (who was likely recommended by a friend, neighbor, or family member in the first place) to make the call on a specialty referral. Of course, the PCP refers each patient to the best specialist in town, right? In reality, this is not the case. No longer do general practitioners "scrub in" to assist surgeons and to personally witness their skill. Primary care referrals are usually based on the physician's past referral experience, friendships, recommendations from other physicians, or political affiliations.

PCPs report that referring a patient to the physician's hospital of choice is only slightly more difficult than referring a patient to a preferred specialist. Patients seem to have stronger opinions about hospitals in their community. Some of these opinions are a function of religious affiliation, perceived technological dominance (particularly with university hospitals), convenient location (for family members and other visitors), hearsay, and personal experience. A 2003 study by VHA found that the most critical indicator of hospital choice among patients is their primary physician's hospital affiliation, followed closely by previous experience, the availability of the needed service, and the advice or referral of a physician. The VHA (2003, 25) study concluded, "When choosing a hospital, consumer considerations are highly subjective and based most often on issues relating to physicians and special clinical needs."

Even in the face of limited but increasing amounts of information about morbidity, mortality, and clinical outcomes, most patients remain totally dependent on their physicians for decisions about their healthcare. The increasing complexity of medical services perpetuates this dependence.

CONCEPT 3: THE RISKS OF PURCHASING HEALTHCARE SERVICES

In the past several decades, business and industry have been preoccupied with the challenge of improving the quality of products and services by reducing variability in the processes used to create those products and services. In the early days of the quality movement, the United States learned difficult lessons from Japanese businesses that willingly and wisely adopted many of W. Edwards Deming's variation-reducing principles and achieved competitive advantage in a burgeoning world market. The race for quality improvement was on. Producers of tangible products and providers of services in many industries jumped on the quality bandwagon and began working diligently to understand their processes and reduce variation to ensure consistent quality.

Thankfully, total quality management and other quality improvement initiatives were also adopted by the healthcare industry. Major initiatives to measure clinical quality and service quality have been undertaken by hospitals, health systems, and medical practices of every size. Some healthcare organizations have had significant success in measuring procedural outcomes in an inpatient or outpatient setting, but measuring the outcomes of cognitive services has proven elusive, particularly in ambulatory settings. Several healthcare organizations have made great strides in reducing clinical variability and medical errors through the use of new technology and protocols. However, those who have done so know that the challenge of reducing procedural and cognitive variability among a single medical staff, let alone across the country, is overwhelming

(Garibaldi 1998). Despite protocols and demonstrated best practices, the inseparability of the service from the service provider creates potential for variability in decisions and service quality among providers of healthcare (Anderson 1993). Particularly in cognitive services, this variability is extremely difficult to identify or measure, let alone reduce.

Physician peers and support staff know, and logic supports the fact, that within most single-specialty groups some variability in clinical capability is present. No two physicians, regardless of similarities in training and experience, provide exactly the same quality of care. In fact, significant variation can be seen within the same practice, depending on the physicians' clinical training, the intensity of peer pressure, past experience, continuing medical education, malpractice risk, and even personal financial motivation. The inseparability of the provider and the service and the resulting variability in care dramatically increase the risk in the customer's healthcare purchasing decision.

That the patient is so personally involved in consuming medical services increases her perceived risk, which is further complicated by the fact that an unsatisfactory outcome cannot be returned or exchanged (Anderson 1993). (The age-old discussion between the chicken and the pig regarding their respective levels of commitment to a ham-and-egg breakfast is illustrative.) The term "going under the knife" certainly conveys the patient's significant personal involvement in the process, and malpractice insurance was developed to assuage the pain and suffering of those with legitimate claims against physicians and hospitals. However, few of those who have experienced poor outcomes as a result of medical errors would likely not trade the monetary compensation they received for a more clinically appropriate result.

Patients' perceived risk influences their behavior as customers in at least three significant ways:

1. *Referrals.* Customers rely heavily on word of mouth when choosing providers. They look for trusted sources of information

about physicians, hospitals, and recommended medical procedures. Based on a review of medical practice data, more than 60 percent of patients select their PCP based on a referral from a friend or relative. The vast majority depend on their PCP for decisions involving a specialist. Despite the availability of data and information about providers in the media and on the Internet, patients prefer and need the counsel of a trusted primary care adviser.

2. *Surrogate measures.* Because most patients do not have the medical knowledge needed to determine the clinical competence of their healthcare providers, they form their opinions based on surrogate measures that have little to do with actual clinical performance. The caring demonstrated by the providers and staff, the convenience or ease of accessing the service, the physical facilities, the wait time, the willingness of the provider to listen and communicate effectively, the quality of food at a facility, and even the way the front-desk staff interact when collecting the patient's copayment are all attributes that are as influential as, and perhaps even more so than, clinical outcomes in defining the patient's customer experience.

3. *Customer loyalty.* According to retail expert Carol Anderson (1993, 175), "a customer's physical involvement in the production of the service can add a deeper level of psychological involvement." Few situations exist in which "physical involvement" is more significant or intimate than in the physician–patient relationship. By its very nature, this relationship requires considerable trust on the part of the patient, who has taken a risk to engage the provider in the first place and who is loathe to change that provider once a relationship is established. At the same time, if the provider violates the patient's trust, the relationship can rarely be rebuilt.

In increasingly competitive markets, PCPs who want to build and maintain successful practices must, intuitively or otherwise, recognize these consumer motivations and behaviors. Physicians must then direct their attention (including adjusting personal attitudes and showing proper behaviors) toward meeting the patients' needs, wants, and priorities as carefully as they address these customers' clinical needs. They must ensure that their office staff go well beyond being nice by seeing to the proper management of the patient/customer's entire experience during each visit. Office policies and procedures must be designed not only to promote high-quality clinical care but also to support quality "caring." Even the physical facility, furnishings, and equipment must be designed around the patient.

Most providers of care in the medical services demand chain—including specialty physicians, hospital departments, and hospital-based specialists—personally interact with the retail customer. As such, they must also each understand and commit to addressing the customer needs, wants, and priorities as fully as they do clinical issues.

Although I am not a clinician and do not have an adequate appreciation of clinical issues, I am a healthcare customer. As such, I understand the customers' attitude toward providers who cannot meet their needs, wants, and priorities: I will take my business elsewhere, and I am not alone.

CONCEPT 4: MAKING YOUR MARKET

What are the implications of these retail concepts for demand chains and their individual members—be they physicians, managers, or staff? The most successful practices, hospitals, and demand chains in competitive environments are those that develop "retail readiness" (Halley 2004).

Retail readiness entails addressing eight areas to ensure that medical care providers understand and meet the needs, wants, and priorities of the customers they want to attract and retain.

1. *Customer knowledge.* How well do we know the needs, wants, and priorities of our current and potential customers? Have

we established systems to solicit this information from customers and potential customers? Do we incorporate current and potential customer feedback into our operating decisions? Is retail customer knowledge shared among demand-chain members?

2. *Customer access.* How convenient are we for customers to access? Do our systems accommodate communication with customers? Are we available when our customers want to see us? Are referrals to other members of the demand chain seamless to our customers?

3. *Customer expectations.* Do we properly influence the perceptions of customers who come to visit us? Do they understand our patient-friendly policies and procedures? Do we help our customers avoid embarrassment and frustration by clearly setting expectations in advance? Are all of our demand-chain members supportive of one another, and do they deliver a consistent service message?

4. *Customer service team.* Given the inseparability of the services delivered by the providers and by the staff, are our team members hired, trained, evaluated, and rewarded for meeting customer needs, wants, and priorities? Do all demand-chain members do their part to ensure a consistent service level?

5. *Customer service culture.* Is high-quality care and caring the expectation within and between demand-chain member organizations? Are poor performers (either providers or staff) moved out of the organization? Are customer complaints carefully analyzed and viewed as opportunities to improve quality and service? Do we periodically audit our retail readiness as demand-chain and individual members? Do we then develop action plans to discuss and correct shortfalls?

6. *Customer service policies.* Are our policies, procedures, and processes customer focused and customer friendly? Or are they geared toward provider convenience or efficient operations?

7. *Education/promotion.* Do we actively and purposely set high customer expectations about our services and the services of other demand-chain members? Do we provide better patient information than our competitors in our offices, through our providers and staff, and on our websites?
8. *Customer experience.* Do we do all we can to ensure that every customer experience is a positive one? Do we ask if we have succeeded? Do we have processes in place to solicit, measure, investigate, and provide feedback on poor performance?

Appendix A (see pages 167–75) shows a retail evaluation questionnaire that was developed to help both primary care and specialty physician offices assess their retail readiness. It is included here for three reasons. First, wise acute care executives will want to foster increasing levels of customer service in their affiliated primary care practices to promote practice development (market share), whether the hospital owns those practices or not. Second, wise specialists and their practice executives will want to ensure that the retail customer's experience in the specialty office will be described to the referring physician in positive terms. Third, to ensure that the retail customer is the center of their collective universe, all demand-chain members will want to make sure that their retail readiness scores are tracked and improving.

Although markets vary significantly around the United States, they share a common fact: they exist in a consumer-choice environment. Customers, even as patients, are more demanding and less tolerant of shoddy service. They are also more appreciative of high-quality service and will be loyal to providers of exceptional service. Quality caring in a medical setting can reduce the risk of malpractice litigation, even in situations where such litigation might be justified. Think about whether your own customer experience validates these statements.

In competitive healthcare markets, those who "make their market" and sustain their competitive advantage do so by focusing on the customer as the center of their universe. The strategies, facilities, technology, staffing, policies, and procedures of these successful organizations and practices ultimately must be shaped by the following filters or questions:

- Will the strategy, facility, technology, staffing, policy, or procedure under consideration positively or negatively affect our ability to deliver high-quality clinical care?
- Will the strategy, facility, technology, staffing, policy, or procedure under consideration positively or negatively affect our understanding of and our ability to meet the needs, wants, and priorities of our retail customers?
- Will the strategy, facility, technology, staffing, policy, or procedure under consideration permit us to remain financially viable so that we can continue to provide the best clinical and service quality?

Those strategies, physicians, policies, technologies, and so on that pass muster will be included in successful demand chains. Those that do not pass the test will be rigorously avoided.

The retail customer is the center of the universe, at least as far as he or she is concerned. Understanding and adapting everything we do to that reality will guarantee competitive advantage and sustainability in increasingly consumer-oriented environments.

NOTES

1. For our purposes, invasive specialties include all the surgical specialties and others whose practices are procedure oriented (e.g., invasive cardiologists). Patients generally do not self-refer to invasive specialists. Noninvasive specialties include those who provide largely cognitive services.

2. The concept of retail customer behavior was originally presented in M. Halley. 2004. "The Case for a Medical Practice Retail Strategy." *The Journal of Medical Practice Management* (November/December): 163–66. Used with permission from Greenbranch Publishing, Phoenix, MD.

REFERENCES

Anderson, C. H. 1993. *Retailing—Concepts, Strategy and Information.* St. Paul, MN: West Publishing Company.

Coile, R. C., Jr. 2002. *Futurescan 2002: A Forecast of Healthcare Trends (2002–2006).* Chicago: Health Administration Press.

Garibaldi, R. A. 1998. "Computers and the Quality of Care—A Clinician's Perspective." *New England Journal of Medicine* 338 (4): 259–60.

Halley, M. D. 2004. "The Case for a Medical Practice Retail Strategy." *Journal of Medical Practice Management* (November/December): 163–66.

VHA. 2003. *Consumers and Health Care: Boomers at the Gate.* Irving, TX: VHA.

CHAPTER 3

The Role of Primary Care Physicians and Other Providers

This chapter presents six concepts:

- Create and keep customers
- Relationship providers versus occurrence providers
- PCP referrals to specialists
- Start-up and growth
- Patient retention
- Customer service as moments of truth

The essence of this chapter is contained in one simple sentence: *Primary care = market share*. For our purposes, market share is the portion of our target population that is captured and retained in our affiliated primary care practices. Although this chapter focuses on primary care physicians or PCPs, and other primary care providers, the concepts discussed here must be clearly understood by all members of the demand chain, including both cognitive and invasive specialists, hospitals, and hospital-based physicians. A clear understanding by all demand-chain members is critical for three reasons.

First, primary care practices feed hospital-based and ambulatory specialty practices as well as hospital inpatient, outpatient, and associated ancillary facilities. The success or failure of every non–primary care member of the demand chain is tied directly to the success of primary care practices at capturing and retaining their (e.g., the hospital's) market share. Hospital executives who understand the primary care business are better able to develop and support the development of PCPs in their primary and secondary markets. This chapter details the principles that drive successful development of primary care practices that are owned or supported by hospitals and multispecialty clinics.

Second, all members of the medical services demand chain come face to face with the ultimate consumer of healthcare services. Consequently, all need to be concerned with developing retail readiness, particularly as it relates to customer service.

Third, the more competitive a particular marketplace is, the more difficult it is for hospitals, specialists, and primary care physicians to remain affiliation-neutral, particularly where their controlling market share is concerned. For healthcare businesses operating in highly competitive environments, to borrow a concept from Roger Blackwell (1997), the battle for competitive dominance and even survival in multisystem markets will be fought among medical services demand chains consisting of affiliated primary care physicians, specialists, hospitals, and hospital-based physicians. And the battle ultimately will be won by demand chains that are successful at capturing market share in primary care practices and attracting that market share to affiliated specialists and directly into affiliated inpatient, outpatient, and ancillary services.

CONCEPT 1: CREATE AND KEEP CUSTOMERS

According to Peter Drucker (2001), the purpose of any organization, particularly in business, is to "create and keep a customer."

Every measurable outcome—from a company's stock value and profitability to the most minute performance ratio—is a function of this primary purpose. Even the loftiest mission statement and the most profound value proposition are irrelevant unless the organization is able to create and keep customers.

I have witnessed numerous debates over whether healthcare in general and ambulatory medical care in particular is a business. In some circles, the use of the term "customer" in place of "patient" is offensive. Vocabulary aside, the point is that a medical practice needs to attract and retain patients or customers to become or remain viable. As in the case with mission statements and financial performance indicators, the greatest clinical skill becomes irrelevant if no one chooses to use clinical services. Primary care physicians—particularly those who have owned their own practices and know what it means to meet a payroll—understand clearly that the medical practice "game" is won or lost on the revenue side of the income statement.

Most private-practice physicians have a keen understanding of the daily patient volumes required to meet payroll and other operating expenses as well as the number of additional patient visits they must schedule to meet their personal financial needs. These private practitioners know without a doubt that the failure to attract and retain enough active patients has dire consequences. Few physicians would use the term "active patient population," but the term, by definition, represents the market share attracted and retained by that particular physician.

CONCEPT 2: RELATIONSHIP PROVIDERS VERSUS OCCURRENCE PROVIDERS

Let's return to Mrs. Smith, who makes most of the healthcare decisions for her family. When she moves to town, she does not select a cardiologist; orthopedic surgeon; gastroenterologist; or an ear, nose, and throat specialist just in case she or a family member requires these services. Unless Mrs. Smith or a family member suffers from a preexisting condition, she will likely select doctors from among four primary care specialties: family medicine, pediatrics, general internal medicine, and obstetrics/gynecology. (She might select an internal medicine/pediatrics physician if she is familiar with this specialty and if such physician is available in her area.)

These primary care specialties and a few internal medicine sub-specialties that treat chronic disease are "relationship providers." In contrast to "occurrence providers," who handle admissions or cases or who provide ancillary testing, relationship providers often see patients several times per year. During these visits, trust can be developed and relationships solidified. Perhaps even more important for the growth and long-term viability of the practice are the referrals that come from adult patients or guardians who are favorably impressed with the physicians and their practice experience. This sales force of satisfied patients is a gold mine and will be discussed later in this chapter.

CONCEPT 3: PCP REFERRALS TO SPECIALISTS

From the perspective of the medical services demand chain, the major role of primary care physicians and other relationship providers is to capture and retain patients. The target patient population is sometimes referred to as market share or a "book of business." The task of capturing market share is best achieved when physicians and other caregivers provide high-quality medical care in a responsive and caring manner.

A second but equally critical role of PCPs is to provide patients appropriate access to medical and surgical specialists, hospital inpatient and outpatient care, and ancillary services providers. From a clinical perspective, PCPs' coordinating role helps to ensure timely access to appropriate services and, when the demand chain functions properly, guarantees continuity of medical care. From the patient's perspective, the PCP serves as a trusted adviser who helps navigate the complexities of selecting a specialty physician, hospital, and ancillary services.

Consider, for example, the 50-year-old male who dutifully sees his general internist for an annual physical. The trusted internist advises her long-time and otherwise healthy patient of a concern noted on the electrocardiogram. A precautionary trip to a cardiologist is recommended. This otherwise healthy male probably has not come to his annual physical having already reviewed performance data for the several dozen cardiologists in town. His anxiety level now elevated, he will likely have three questions for his internist: (1) Which cardiologist do you want me to see? (2) How soon can we make an appointment? (3) Is the recommended cardiologist on my insurance panel?

One of the questions my consultant team and I routinely ask PCPs is how easily they are able to refer patients to their (the PCPs') specialist of choice. The majority of physicians confirm that their patients rely on them to recommend their (the PCPs') preferred specialists. They generally report that, nine times out of ten, patients accept the specialty referral without question.

Experience has shown that the traditional gatekeeper concept, which placed on primary care providers the burden of restricting access to care, was flawed. But out of that concept managed care companies brought to light the tremendous influence that PCPs have on the flow of referrals. For years, enlightened and successful specialists in communities across the United States have built and maintained relationships to attract primary care referrals. As managed care and capitation loomed on the horizon, hospitals also recognized the referral potential and acquired primary care practices by the hundreds.

Unfortunately, instead of entering the business of primary care with the intent of being successful in that business, most hospitals treated the medical practices they owned like any other department of the hospital, ignoring the rules for success. (McDonald's and Ruth's Chris Steak House are both restaurants, but the rules for success in one do not apply to the other.) The results were financially and politically disastrous for many, and by the late 1990s divestiture became the trend across the healthcare landscape. Many hospitals and health systems eliminated or pruned their primary care networks. Others starved their networks by failing to properly capitalize on them. Frequently, the best physicians left first. If they went back to private practice or to a competitor within the community, their patients followed. Otherwise, their patient populations dissipated.

By the early 2000s I began receiving calls from hospitals and health systems, particularly in competitive markets, that were alert enough to notice the decline in throughput that seemed to correlate with their divestiture of primary care practices. I was not surprised, of course, because in terminating their relationship with primary care physicians, they had also divested their market share. The hospitals suffered, and some of their affiliated specialists had to start working at competing facilities to survive.

CONCEPT 4: START-UP AND GROWTH

Primary care is market share, and capturing that market share—whether for offensive or defensive purposes—is a prime survival imperative for every member of the medical services demand chain, particularly hospitals. Given the critical nature of this directive, understanding how primary care practices evolve is vital, and their development must not be left to chance. Having observed or managed the start-up of several new hospital-owned or hospital-supported primary care practices over the years, I recommend that a new primary care physician attempting to capture market share consider the following three factors.

Appropriate Location

One of the first rules of good retailing is "location, location, location." Unless you are also planning to sell gas, cigarettes, and beer, your primary care practice does not need to be located at a busy street corner, with ingress and egress on both sides, or near a stoplight. Choosing the right geographic location, however, is particularly critical in "cold starts." A cold start is a new practice started by a new or experienced physician in a new location without the benefit of an established partner. What location factors are important for physicians planning to open their own new practices or for hospitals implementing their retail strategy?

First, in an urban or suburban setting, convenience is a key consideration in Mrs. Smith's selection of a primary care provider. Based on the zip code analyses we have performed for numerous primary care practices, we have found that patients tend to select a PCP within a reasonable distance of their place of residence. Frequently, this means less than five miles or a ten-minute drive from home. A new primary care office must be located in a growing market with adequate numbers of potential customers to support existing primary care practices and the new physician. Few things are more devastating to a new physician and his staff (or potentially costly to a physician or hospital owner) than mistakenly locating in a market area that cannot support additional provider capacity.

Second, the selected office location will dramatically influence the patient profile and the payer mix that will ultimately be attracted by the practice. For example, a federally qualified community health center that targets the needs of the medically underserved must be located within an easy drive or along bus routes to facilitate patient access. Likewise, those practices desiring a high-end payer mix will want to locate in or near areas where the average household income is consistent with the patient population and payer mix sought by the physician or as a part of the hospital's market-share objectives.

Effective Physician Communication and Interpersonal Skills

Over the years it has become easier for me to recognize physician personalities that are likely to build a strong practice. One trait that particularly stands out is the ability to communicate effectively. An effective communicator is able to listen attentively, reflect understanding, and convey caring. Patients assume, correctly or otherwise, that physicians are clinically competent. Clinical competence is important to patients, but they equally value a physician's ability to communicate. This factor is critical to hospitals and/or medical practices involved in recruiting new providers to a community. Clinical training and board eligibility or certification are important but are not enough to ensure the development of a busy practice. A pleasant and engaging personality is essential.

Ability to Develop a "Sales Force"

Every successful PCP knows by experience that her practice has developed and remains viable through word of mouth from one satisfied patient to another. Primary care practices that track the sources of their new patients often find that more than 60 percent of new patient volume can be attributed to a personal referral from a friend or relative. The next highest source of referrals is often the Yellow Pages directory, which usually accounts for less than 20 percent of new patient business.

Certainly, practice development can be kick-started by the "grand opening" of a new practice or the addition of a new physician to an established practice. Direct-mail campaigns to local neighborhoods will also attract some unattached customers. However, the natural development process cannot be short-circuited. Hospitals in particular are often disappointed that their heavy advertising expenditures do not boost a new practice as expected. Advertising campaigns are valuable, but the development of a core group of satisfied patients who refer friends and relatives is what ultimately determines success or failure. This passive "sales force" does not develop quickly or geometrically. It develops slowly over time through consistent caring performance by the physician and all staff members.

As a result of this natural development process, most cold-start practices take a minimum of 18, and usually 24, months to reach maturity. Using average patient visits per physician per day as a performance measure, a cold-start practice can be projected to reach 40–45 percent of capacity, as a run rate, by month 12 and 85–90 percent of capacity by month 24. The only ways in which I have seen this two-year development cycle successfully shortened are by (1) locating the new physician in a group practice with other established providers, (2) having the new physician take over the practice of a retiring physician, and (3) placing the new physician in a market with significant excess demand.

The patients of established partners provide a ready-made sales force for referring new patients to the practice, and these new patients can be directed to the new provider. Some attrition will occur when a new provider takes over the practice of a retiring physician, but the majority of the patients will usually remain with the practice if the new physician has good communication skills. Referral momentum also is created when significant excess demand exists for primary care services in a particular community or market area. In addition, practices with female PCPs often experience rapid growth in markets where there is a lack of women providers. In each of these cases, word of mouth still drives practice viability.

CONCEPT 5: PATIENT RETENTION

Let's return to Peter Drucker's assertion that the purpose of any organization is to create and keep a customer. Because even the newest primary care practice is absolutely dependent on referrals from satisfied patients, customer retention is a critical priority from the start. Fortunately, experience has shown that once Mrs. Smith selects and is comfortable with her PCP, she is loathe to change. This is great news for primary care providers who are the first to enter a market. For those who attempt to enter saturated markets, it presents a potentially insurmountable challenge. This precept should capture the attention of every hospital strategist considering market-share acquisition and protection.

Several common barriers to patient retention exist. Payers are the first barrier cited by most physicians, but in recent years the influence of payers on patient migration has lessened. In fact, in most competitive markets today, payers prefer to be inclusive rather than exclusive in selecting a panel of PCPs, thus enhancing their ability to attract more covered lives and premium dollars. The threat always exists that a provider will be dropped by a managed care plan or that practice or hospital-owner strategists will choose to no longer participate with poorly reimbursing plans. In either case, the result is the exodus of a block of patients from the practice. However, these situations tend to be the exception rather than the rule. Most practices have both gains and losses during annual open-enrollment periods, and those adjustments tend to neutralize each other.

Another threat to retention, which is often noted by physicians and administrators, is a new facility built by competitors. A new facility is attractive to some patients; beautiful surroundings, new equipment, or a big name will attract a certain segment of the population. However, existing practices do not necessarily empty out when the local competing hospital builds a new ambulatory care center or when Mayo puts a primary care site in a community. The segment of the population influenced by the size or perceived prestige of such a facility is far from the majority.

The addition of new PCPs to a particular market area is certainly a reason for concern on the part of established physicians, particularly if their practices are too busy or their customer service is lacking (an issue that is addressed in Concept 6). If the new physician offers a unique opportunity to the marketplace, concern should be heightened. For example, if the new physician is a personable female in a male-dominated market area, she will likely take some of that market share, given that women are the major purchasers of healthcare and many women would prefer to receive their healthcare from a female physician. Similarly, if the new physician is a former small-town football hero returning home to practice medicine after many years of training, he will have a unique draw in the community, at least initially.

Once again, however, it is unlikely even in these circumstances that any single, established primary care practice will be devastated in the short run. In fact, in growing market areas, established practices always have an advantage over new practices because of their larger sales force—that is, patients who refer new patients. Obviously, in stagnant markets most practices are hurt when the supply of PCPs exceeds the demand for those services, increasing the potential for the practice to fail and to become vulnerable to acquisition by competitors.

The most significant threats to patient or customer retention are internal and can be divided into two general categories: access and customer service. Access issues include physician availability, physician timeliness, and call coverage.

Physician Availability

As in most other professional practices, the constraining factor in a medical practice is time, as reflected in the appointment schedule. The most successful practices and the most productive physicians pay particular attention to their appointment schedule and tailor it to meet the needs, wants, and priorities of their patients as well as their own practice style. In addition to determining the days they will work and whether they will have early morning or evening hours, successful PCPs must continually look to improve the way in which individual patients are scheduled within those time frames. Time blocks should be scheduled based on patients' primary medical complaint or anticipated procedures. Some physicians use a wave schedule or modified wave schedule to mix and match short appointments with long appointments. Others have transitioned to an open access or advanced access model to ensure that all patients are seen on a same-day basis.

These scheduling models and approaches must be carefully matched to the physician's practice style to ensure that the second measure of accessibility—physician timeliness—is not violated.

Physician Timeliness

Once a schedule is established and patient expectations are set, the practice must do all it can to stay on schedule. Assuming the physician is on time to start the day, it is the clinical assistant who often must keep the practice on schedule.

Next to providing high-quality caring—that is, clinical excellence coupled with compassion—a clinical assistant's most important role is to manage the productivity of the expensive physician resource. The obvious components of this responsibility include keeping the exam rooms occupied, maintaining a useful workup that lists each patient's chief medical complaint, and being available whenever the physician opens an exam-room door. Less obvious is the nuance of understanding how long the physician should be in the exam room to deal with a particular medical complaint and knowing when to slip in to relieve the physician when the patient wants to chat. Obviously, the practice must be organized and staffed in such a way that the clinical assistant can fulfill these responsibilities without getting tied up making telephone calls, which should be delegated to someone else.

Call Coverage

The final component of accessibility is coverage when the physician of choice is not available. The advantage clearly goes to small group practices whose providers have relatively homogeneous practice styles, philosophies, and training. Patients recognize that their preferred provider cannot possibly be available 24/7. At the same time, patients prefer being able to reach a physician who will respond in a reasonably similar manner. Naturally, access to the patient's medical history, most recent visit, and current medications facilitates this preferred behavior by the covering physician. A well-implemented electronic medical record enhances the covering physician's ability, both clinically and from a customer service perspective.

All three of these factors affect contract considerations for new employed physicians, whether the employer is a group practice or a hospital. An employed physician's office schedule, a productivity compensation model, and call coverage requirements should all be defined carefully to promote patient access.

CONCEPT 6: CUSTOMER SERVICE AS MOMENTS OF TRUTH

Ultimately, the key to creating and keeping a customer in a primary care practice—or in any healthcare setting—is a customer service experience that meets or exceeds the patient's expectations. For this reason, the top priority for successful physicians, their managers, and support staff should be to ensure a positive experience for each customer, each day. A high level of customer service captures the new patients that come through the door and retains the established patient population. These satisfied patients become a natural sales force yielding additional customers.

Why do some practices, departments, and networks excel at delivering high-quality care and caring while others languish in mediocrity? The answer is that too many organizations leave customer service to chance, with little more than an occasional patient satisfaction survey and instructions for everyone to "be nice." Successful practices build caring into their culture. They hire for it, talk about it, and insist on it as a condition of continued employment. Neither physicians nor management nor staff tolerate insensitive or inconsiderate behavior on the part of team members. (These same principles apply to specialty practices, and the concepts are easily modified for the hospital and hospital-based physicians, whether the customer is the retail patient or the referring physician.)

Many customer service training programs, aimed largely at hospitals and occasionally at medical practices, have been successful at reminding physicians, support staff, and management about the importance of maintaining a high level of customer service and at measuring and improving the level of service. Unfortunately, unless these occasional booster shots are accompanied by an ingrained customer service culture, their effectiveness quickly fades under the pressure of busy offices or departments and established routines.

Lessons from an Airline

In a wonderful treatise on developing a customer service culture, Jan Carlzon, former president and CEO of Scandinavian Air Systems (SAS), describes his company's emphasis on "moments of truth" (Carlzon 1987). When Carlzon first became president of SAS, it was a cash-strapped regional carrier struggling to maintain its place against much larger and financially well-heeled competitors. Constrained by limited capital resources, Carlzon carefully targeted business travelers as his most likely source of consistent revenue. He knew that to capture and retain this highly sought-after customer, he had to develop a sustainable advantage in the face of stiff competition. He knew that competing on price would not be a sustainable competitive approach, given the deep pockets of the other carriers. Instead, he looked for a way to focus his entire organization on meeting the needs, wants, and priorities of rushed and often weary travelers. He knew that the keys to success included multiple flights to key cities and on-time departures and arrivals. Even more importantly, he realized that if he developed a culture that could meet or exceed each traveler's expectations, larger competitors would have a difficult time matching SAS's service outcomes.

To achieve such high levels of service, Carlzon and his team examined travelers' experiences and identified the key moments when travelers came into contact with SAS personnel. Managing these moments of truth to meet or exceed customer expectations then became an organization-wide focus. Just as important, Carlzon recognized that meeting customer expectations at each moment of truth would require local, even individual, authority to act in a timely manner—at the moment of truth. He understood that management's role was to ensure that employees who handle these critical moments were properly trained and that barriers to their success—including long-standing but outmoded policies and procedures—were removed. Although risky, Carlzon's vision and the efforts of SAS employees paid off. In 1994, just months after Carlzon took the helm, SAS was voted Airline of the Year by *Air Transport World*.

I have worked with several organizations in applying Carlzon's concepts to a particular practice, department, or service line. These participants do not take more than a few minutes to identify the moments of truth experienced by patients/customers in their particular setting. In a primary care office, for example, the list may include the following moments of truth during which a new patient touches and forms an impression about the practice (again, these moments are illustrative of the retail setting and can be modified for specialists and hospital departments):

1. *Referral.* The majority of new patients come to a practice as a result of a referral from a friend or relative. The referral process begins to establish the new patient's expectations. Naturally, the "salesperson" making the referral will likely describe the practice in terms of his own positive experience with the physician and staff (hence, the critical role of exceptional customer service).

2. *Initial contact.* The patient's initial contact tends to confirm or refute the expectations established by the salesperson. Practices that focus attention on meeting a patient's first or second request for an appointment and that continually measure their performance are more likely to succeed at this important moment of truth.

3. *Welcome packet.* If the patient requests a complete physical, a slight delay is likely between the initial contact and the appointment. Some practices take advantage of this delay and mail a welcome packet containing such information as a letter from the physician, a map, a brochure, selected health information, and a health history form that can be completed before the first visit. If the visit request is more acute,

the welcome packet may be sent out after the first visit, with appropriate modifications.

4. *Reception.* One of the most critical opportunities to meet patient expectations occurs at the reception desk. Unfortunately, in many practices receptionists spend a great deal of their time doing anything but receiving patients. Physical barriers, such as small reception windows or a glass partition, communicate something other than the welcome that retail customers expect from those who supposedly understand their needs, wants, and priorities. Hiring the right reception staff and removing physical barriers to an appropriate welcome should be top priorities.

5. *Reception room.* No practice should have a "waiting room." Although it is sometimes necessary, waiting adds no value to the customer's experience. Consequently, wait time should be kept to a minimum and should be carefully managed to ensure that the patient is as comfortable as possible. In some practices, the waiting room can become a black hole, offering little opportunity for escape. The classic reason for this black hole is that the receptionist thinks her job is complete once the patient is checked in and the chart is placed in the clinical assistant's box. The clinical assistant, of course, is usually busy with other patients or on the phone and does not know how long the patient has been waiting. In reality, the receptionist's responsibility for each patient should not end until that patient is called into the exam room by the clinical assistant. Receptionists should be encouraged to act like lifeguards, watching for each head bobbing in the reception area, tracking wait times, and managing patients' expectations about when they will be seen. These are critical receptionist duties in a practice concerned about the needs, wants, and priorities of its customers. Signs such as one that reads "If you've been waiting more than 20 minutes, please check with the receptionist" would never be found in a practice that is focused on the customer.

6. *The clinical assistant.* The clinical assistant in a primary care practice has two interrelated and critical roles. The first is to provide high-quality care and caring. The second is to manage the physician's productivity. The clinical assistant's watch begins when he calls the patient from the reception room into the clinical area. Consider the following tasks performed by a clinical assistant:

- Greeting the patient
- Noting vital signs and chief complaint
- Instructing the patient to change into a gown as needed
- Managing the patient's expectations and comfort while in the exam room
- Attaching relevant health information to the medical chart that can be delivered to the patient by the physician
- Monitoring the physician's time spent in the exam room and "slipping in" as appropriate to move the physician on to the next patient
- Providing guidance about ancillary services ordered by the physician
- Instructing the patient about specialty referrals as needed
- Getting the patient dressed and back down the hall to the front desk

The clinical assistant often performs these activities in multiple exam rooms while also occasionally helping the physician in minor procedures such as laceration repair.

The clinical assistant's role is without a doubt essential. Unfortunately, clinical assistants are often found on the telephone (e.g., making referral calls) or performing nonclinical duties that can and should be delegated to others. Often the most productive and service-oriented physicians require more than one clinical assistant to accomplish the critical dual roles of providing high-quality care and caring and managing the physician's productivity.

7. *Ancillary services.* Laboratory and radiology services offered in the office provide tremendous convenience and another opportunity to retain the customer. One-stop shops are preferred over practices that require patients to exit and travel, even down the hall, for ancillary procedures that could be performed in the primary care office. For patients requiring ancillary services, the handoff from the clinical assistant to the ancillary service technician must be flawless. Again, the wait time must be kept to a minimum, and the ancillary service technician must be well trained, confident, and caring.

8. *The exit.* Exiting the practice is often poorly handled simply because this moment of truth is not perceived to be as critical as the clinical experience. However, in the patient's mind, the exit process is crucial. Patients want privacy and an appropriate response from a cashier regarding copays (which may have been handled by the receptionist), deductibles, and insurance questions. This is particularly true for patients who do not understand medical insurance—knowledge that most cashiers take for granted. Making sure that the process of collecting at the point of service, responding effectively to the patient's reimbursement questions, and scheduling any follow-up appointments goes smoothly is absolutely critical to the entire experience. The exit requires the same level of personal interest and caring as any moment of truth in the clinical experience.

9. *Billing.* One of the greatest potential sources of frustration for patients is the billing process. Every office involved in the billing process knows that the number of telephone calls from confused or frustrated patients increases dramatically in the first few days after statements are mailed. Successful practices are concerned about improving the clarity of patient statements to reduce the level of frustration and the potential for misunderstanding. They also recognize that, despite their best efforts, patients will still have questions about statements and insurance claims. However, successful practices view these phone calls as opportunities to provide a valuable service and to continue

demonstrating the caring philosophy the patient experienced during his visit. Even precollection activities should reflect a caring attitude. Patients should always be given the benefit of the doubt and treated with the greatest of respect.

Moments of truth receive constant attention in successful primary care practices, specialty offices, and hospital departments. Each moment requires a clear understanding of patient expectations, the establishment of performance standards, the assignment of responsibility, the monitoring of performance, the review of feedback, and the placing of accountability for outcomes. Moments of truth generally provide ample fodder for weekly department meetings and monthly all-staff discussions. Only consistent attention to these details by physicians, management, and staff will yield the kind of culture change that is required to meet the needs, wants, and priorities of patients. The payoff, however, can be phenomenal.

REFERENCES

Blackwell, R. D. 1997. *From Mind to Market—Reinventing the Retail Supply Chain.* New York: HarperCollins.

Carlzon, J. 1987. *Moments of Truth—New Strategies for Today's Customer-Driven Economy.* Cambridge, MA: Ballinger Publishing Company.

Drucker, P. F. 2001. *The Essential Drucker.* New York: HarperCollins.

CHAPTER 4

The Role of Specialists

This chapter presents four concepts:

- Two personal anecdotes
- Technician or healer?
- The retail customer and the specialist
- Primary care providers as customers

From the hospital CEO's perspective, non–hospital-based specialty physicians wear a number of significant and sometimes conflicting hats. They are certainly customers, who are often responsible for millions of dollars in hospital revenue. They are members or officers of the medical staff. They may be medical directors of key programs or service lines. Specialists may also be hospital employees and even hospital board members, or they may be competitors who have built ambulatory surgery or diagnostic centers.

Regardless of their relationship with the hospital or the hat they wear at a particular time, specialty physicians play a key role in attracting market share to the hospitals with whom they choose to affiliate. As such, the success or failure of specialty practices and their physicians has a direct impact on the success of the hospital and the entire demand chain.

Hospital and specialty group executives who recruit and support these highly trained physicians must understand what role specialists play and how specialists can be effective members of the demand chain. Developing the right mix of specialties, recruiting the right physicians for that mix, and ensuring the success of those practices should be the interest of every hospital CEO. This chapter details the principles behind successful specialty practices and physicians who make ideal demand-chain members.

CONCEPT 1: TWO PERSONAL ANECDOTES

Kaden's Story

Two personal anecdotes illustrate many of the key topics in this chapter. The first involves my grandson, Kaden, who was born with a tracheoesophageal fistula (TEF) and esophageal atresia, a condition in which the esophagus and trachea fail to develop properly and the bottom portion of the esophagus that rises from the stomach becomes attached to the trachea or windpipe. The top portion of the esophagus, finding no connection, closes at the bottom, giving the appearance of a small thumb hanging from the back of the throat.

Kaden's unusual condition was discovered by skilled nurses and was confirmed by a well-prepared neonatologist in the hospital where he was born. Within hours, he was transferred to the regional hospital, where they deal with several cases of this condition each year. Fortunately, the surgeon on call not only was technically skilled but also provided clear information about the condition, the surgical options, and the potential outcomes. This busy surgeon took out a pen and drew pictures of the condition and potential surgical repair for a young, naturally distraught father and an appreciative grandfather. The surgeon then went on to apply his skills and repair the anomaly using the appropriate technology.

Twenty-nine days later—with several physicians, nurse practitioners, nurses, and other caring individuals as new friends—Kaden came home. One of the common challenges for TEF babies is the development of significant acid reflux; Kaden proved not exempt from this challenge. From the first days of his life, Kaden was taking adult doses of acid reflux medication. Despite minor challenges, Kaden thrived for several months. Shortly before his first birthday, however, he began having unexplained choking spells, some of which were so serious that he passed out. These spells became more frequent, and he was admitted again to the regional hospital for further testing.

After several uneventful days in the hospital, my daughter, Andrea, was told that she would likely be able to bring Kaden home. Later that same day, however, a nurse practitioner informed her that Kaden would be scheduled for surgery, providing no explanation other than the name of the procedure. Naturally, Andrea was upset and confused. I assured her that no one would perform surgery on her child without her authorization and that she should not sign any documents until she had a clear understanding of the reason, the risks, and the potential outcomes of the procedure.

Andrea talked with the nurse assigned to Kaden that evening, and the nurse was kind enough to find some literature on the particular procedure mentioned by the nurse practitioner. Unfortunately, this literature heightened Andrea's concern. Andrea was told that Kaden's primary surgeon was out of town and that his partner would come the following morning to provide further detail about the procedure.

Andrea's previous experience with this partner was not positive. She found him to be insensitive and impatient, and she felt he spoke down to her. I promised her I would come to the hospital to meet with her and this surgeon.

The next morning, when the surgeon entered the room, we were waiting with our questions. Andrea started the conversation by explaining to him that she was uncomfortable with her level of understanding of the procedure, its potential lifetime implications for her son, and the practical implications of the gastrostomy tube, or "g-tube," she was told would be protruding from his stomach for months or years. The surgeon was informed that Andrea refused to sign any paperwork, and he seemed exasperated by our need for more information. His curt response about the need for the surgery was, "If he doesn't have the surgery, he will die." He further explained that Kaden would not be able to drink soda pop or eat spicy foods because the surgery would likely result in the inability to burp or vomit—hence, the need for the g-tube. We were also informed that this surgeon had done several of these procedures, information that did not sway us nor did it set our minds at ease about the surgeon or the procedure.

On at least two more occasions later that day, we were asked to sign the paperwork. We again explained that we would not be signing the paperwork until Andrea had a chance to visit with her primary surgeon, who was scheduled to return the next day. We were very frustrated.

Fortunately, Kaden's original surgeon returned to work the following day. He visited Andrea and Kaden first thing that morning, the same day the surgery had been scheduled. He sat down with Andrea and carefully explained the reason he felt the surgery was necessary, discussed the procedure itself, how he would tailor the outcome to Kaden's particular needs, and the potential lifelong implications for this one-year-old child. During this visit, he spoke to Kaden and stroked his hair. Before leaving, he made sure all of Andrea's questions and concerns were addressed. He was realistic about the risks and expressed his belief that the procedure would help improve the quality of Kaden's life. At the conclusion of their discussion, Andrea indicated she was comfortable giving permission for the procedure. The entire discussion took little more than ten minutes—about the same amount of time the less-sensitive partner had spent the day before.

What made the difference? Was it perceived clinical competence? Was it a clinically accurate description of the procedure? Was it the threat of the dire consequence if the surgery was not performed? It was none of these. The simple reason Andrea's entire disposition changed toward the medical procedure can be summarized in the words she shared with me shortly after the surgeon's departure: "He cares about my baby."

This experience is a testimony to anyone interested in developing a successful specialty practice. At the same time, it is an indictment of those specialists who lose their perspective and become little more than competent technicians.

The Optometrist

The second anecdote is about an incident that occurred some years ago, when I visited my optometrist for a long overdue eye examination and an updated prescription. The optometrist dilated my eyes and provided a complete exam. Noting what is termed "lattice degeneration," he suggested that I visit an ophthalmologist to determine whether a laser procedure might be required. One of my clients at the time was an ophthalmologist who specialized in laser surgery. I asked if my optometrist had ever referred a patient to this ophthalmologist in a city some 35 miles south. He indicated that he had not done so but would be happy to accommodate my request.

At the time of my referral, there was tremendous animosity between optometrists and ophthalmologists in that state over the issue of prescriptive privileges. Arguments were being made at the state legislature, and the ugliness that sometimes accompanies such battles had spilled over into the local press.

At the appointed day and time, I arrived at the ophthalmologist's office, where I was greeted warmly and ushered into an examination room. My eyes were once again dilated. Several minutes later, the ophthalmologist entered and greeted me warmly. What occurred over the next few minutes helped me understand why this specialist had such a large referral following among optometrists and other ophthalmologists.

In examining my eye, he encountered the lattice degeneration and complimented my optometrist, by name, for correctly diagnosing the problem. Using a phone in the exam room, he asked his assistant to place a call to my optometrist to discuss my situation. Within a few minutes, the exam-room phone rang and the optometrist was connected with the ophthalmologist.

At that point, the ophthalmologist did three critical things. First, he again indicated to the optometrist, in my presence, that the diagnosis was accurate. Second, he engaged the optometrist in a discussion of a proposed treatment plan, even asking for his opinion. Third, at the conclusion of their discussion, the ophthalmologist said, "I will send Mr. Halley back to you for follow-up." Is it any wonder that this ophthalmologist had one of the most successful practices in the region?

These two anecdotes provide a context for the principles that govern the success of individual specialty physicians and their impact on the success of the entire demand chain.

CONCEPT 2: TECHNICIAN OR HEALER?

During the past few decades, medical research and technical advances have dramatically increased the complexity and capabilities of medical science. Educators have responded by increasing the depth and specialization of medical training programs. One criticism of this increased specialization and technical complexity is the relatively narrow scope of procedural alternatives likely to be considered by a given specialist. An orthopedic surgeon, for example, might legitimately recommend a surgical procedure, whereas a physical medicine and rehabilitation physician might initially recommend a more conservative approach. The clinical debate about which physician is "right" involves a number of variables, including medical judgment, and will be resolved only by years of careful outcomes measurement. A similar debate has raged over the use of stents implanted by cardiologists versus the more invasive bypass alternative provided by cardiovascular surgeons. Again, only time and careful outcomes measurement will resolve the debate.

Regardless of the clinical questions and outcomes, a more fundamental question has emerged: Has increased specialization, with its attendant technical benefits, turned physicians/healers, who practice both the art and the science of medicine, into highly skilled technicians? The answer goes well beyond the clinical issues to each specialty physician's motivation to understand and meet the needs, wants, and priorities of patients/customers and of referring physicians/customers. Simply put, "healers" care enough to understand needs, wants, and priorities. "Technicians" are too busy to provide the caring along with the medical care. My daughter's comment about my grandson's surgeon says it all: "He cares about my baby."

For even the most gifted and caring physician, being a caring provider in the face of today's medical practice realities is a monumental task. The continued downward pressure on reimbursement, the ever-present threat of malpractice lawsuits, increased regulation and more aggressive enforcement, increasing labor costs and malpractice premiums, and other trends have forever changed the face of medical care delivery. Even with the addition of certain ancillary services, often facilitated by improved technology, many physicians have had to increase the volume of patients (to whom they provide both cognitive and invasive services) to maintain financially viable practices while continuing to draw market-competitive compensation. Private-practice specialists, in particular, are painfully aware of the daily, weekly, and monthly patient volumes and charges they must generate to maintain viable businesses and to continue providing high-quality medical care. Despite relatively high incomes, very few specialists can afford to practice medicine as a hobby.

Naturally, the drive for increased patient volume and the limited number of hours in a day reduce the amount of time physicians can spend understanding and meeting patients' needs, wants, and priorities.

In addition to serving patients effectively, specialists must also be mindful of the needs, wants, and priorities of those PCPs and others from whom they receive referrals. These referral customers are just as vital to the success of a specialty practice as are the patients themselves. I have worked with specialists who were technically superb but were inept when it came to building and maintaining relationships with referring physicians. I have often been engaged by anxious hospital executives who were fearful of losing specialists who were unable to build a sustainable practice volume. One neurologist, for example, painstakingly reviewed with me his extensive training and clinical background, indicating that his peers on the medical staff ought to recognize his clinical superiority. Fortunately, his support staff had carefully tracked the source of each patient referral since the beginning of the practice nearly two years earlier. A computerized report clearly demonstrated a pattern of PCPs and others referring patients over a few months and then abruptly stopping. In fact, of those physicians who referred patients during the first year, very few appeared on the second-year report. Based on feedback from patients and physicians, the neurologists' office manager and staff uncovered the practice's challenges. The neurologist had a difficult time communicating verbally with his physician referral sources. Patients perceived him as abrasive and aloof, and they communicated their feelings to their referring physician. That feedback, of course, was the death knell for the practice. Despite attempted interventions, the neurologist ended up going to work in a salaried position for a staff-model health maintenance organization where referring physicians and patients had no other alternatives.

CONCEPT 3: THE RETAIL CUSTOMER AND THE SPECIALIST

Economists use the term "utility" to help describe consumer behavior in meeting their own self-interest. Utility in this context is the level of satisfaction or perceived value derived from a decision to purchase a particular good or service. An office visit to a PCP may have relatively low utility for some patients. No-shows routinely leave gaping holes in a provider's schedule, especially on nice summer days when everyone would rather be doing something other than waiting in an exam room. Smart PCPs often have their staff members call patients who have scheduled longer appointments for annual physicals and diagnostic procedures just to make sure they show up. Others have considered charging a fee to patients who fail to show up for an appointment or dismissing repeat offenders from the practice.

When a PCP refers a retail customer to a specialist, anecdotal experience (and logic) indicates that the utility of the specialty visit increases for the patient—sometimes dramatically. Rather than going to the doctor for a routine visit or test, the patient/customer is now "real sick" or "real hurt." Patient anxiety is often heightened with a referral to a specialist. Something may be seriously wrong, even life threatening. This increased utility results in the following dynamics:

- *No shows.* The no-show rate for specialty practices drops, especially for initial consultations and visits.
- *Referral influence.* Patients are more easily directed to the specialist chosen by their trusted PCP, even if that specialist is across town, against traffic-migration patterns, and affiliated with a different hospital.
- *Access.* Patient anxiety (and sometimes PCP anxiety) is heightened, making the timeliness of the visit paramount.
- *Caring.* In addition to high-quality clinical care, sicker patients, more anxious patients, and postsurgical patients are naturally less tolerant and more sensitive to their physician-office experience. They require a higher level of sensitivity and care than their relatively healthy counterparts in primary care offices.
- *Information.* Control of our environment and circumstances is a natural human need. A physical malfunction is a significant disrupter of our perceived control. Consequently, our need for information is critical, as is our participation in decisions affecting our current and future health.

- *Relative compliance.* Logic suggests, and anecdotal evidence confirms, that compliance with specialist-recommended treatment is higher than with primary care services because of the potentially more serious consequences of failing to comply.

The implications of these dynamics for specialty physicians are obvious.

I have heard it said, "They don't care how much you know until they know how much you care." This may be a trite statement, but it is true. As mentioned earlier, caring requires time. It requires an understanding of patient needs, wants, and priorities. It requires a consistent effort to ensure that the entire patient experience adds to, rather than detracts from, meeting the patient's expectations.

In most offices, the responsiveness at the appointment desk sets the tone for the entire patient experience. A welcome package with a note from the doctor, clear directions to the office, and a reasonable set of professionally printed paperwork contribute to a positive first impression. The physical location and facilities with appropriate professional ambience add to the experience. The warmth of a receptionist who greets and helps each patient get settled in a reception room (not the "black hole" waiting room found in some offices) is essential to the process. (By the way, sliding glass windows separating the receptionist from the reception area are not conducive to the warm greeting or the reception-room management required of an effective receptionist. Yes, I have heard all of the arguments about confidentiality behind the front desk. Sometimes I fear we forget we exist to serve the patients rather than the regulators. Get rid of the glass!)

Receptionists who act like lifeguards keep track of every bobbing head in the reception room and hand off each patient to the clinical assistant. That handoff is best made to a smiling and sensitive nurse or medical assistant who calls the patient by name, carries on an age-appropriate conversation, and escorts the patient to the examination room. This caring professional then listens closely to the issue(s) at hand and prepares the patient, the room, and the chart so that the physician can efficiently and effectively meet the patient's clinical needs as well as the patient's reasonable wants and priorities. Although the physician manages the patient's clinical needs, an effective clinical assistant is in the best position to manage the patient's expectations about the visit and the doctor. The clinical assistant also can slip into the exam room and take over when a patient just wants to chat.

Naturally, the physician's interaction with the patient is critical. The patient needs to be heard, to feel understood, and to be educated regarding the medical condition, testing and treatment, and the attendant risks. As illustrated in the anecdote about my grandson, the time it takes to accomplish these critical tasks is less an issue than the caring attitude of the physician (and any assistants). "He cares about my baby" are words that will ring in my ears forever! Providing clear verbal information, drawings, and literature is also essential. Why let the Internet or television educate our patients regarding their conditions when neither provides a medical chart or a physical examination?

Of course, postexamination ancillary services, procedure scheduling, and follow-up appointments must be handled with equal caring to ensure a consistently positive patient experience. The billing process is a critical part of this experience. The attitude required of all those working with patients and their guarantors is to assist the patient with helping the practice get paid for its high-quality services. The billing office exists to serve the patient and advocate for the patient with insurance carriers and with the practice. Billing professionals must assume that most patients are honorable and want to see their physician paid fairly. Otherwise, the insurance and private-pay receivables management process can destroy a flawless patient experience.

CONCEPT 4: PRIMARY CARE PROVIDERS AS CUSTOMERS

I have witnessed many new PCPs start new medical practices. Others have joined established group practices where they have benefited from reduced start-up risks, an established practice infrastructure, and overflow from established patients. When new physicians start a practice, especially when they relocate to a new community, they often select specialists in the same way that Mrs. Smith selects her PCP. They ask a neighbor, usually one of their associates, who she uses for orthopedics, dermatology, general surgery, and other specialties. Naturally, the associate will recommend the specialists that she has used successfully.

And what does "used successfully" mean? If PCPs referred only to the most clinically competent specialist in town, one doctor would be busy and the rest would go hungry. Lining up all 14 cardiologists in the community and asking PCPs to identify the most clinically competent specialist would likely yield a variety of opinions and answers rather than a definitive "best." In most of the strategic planning retreats that my colleagues and I have facilitated over the years, the groups with whom we have worked have all claimed to have the "best" physicians in the marketplace—until asked to justify that response. Very few organizations can prove that they have the best physicians, especially among the more cognitive specialties. (Outliers, whose clinical reputation is beyond question, certainly exist, but most specialists do not fall into this category.) In communities where a technical-best physician has been identified in a certain specialty, others within that same specialty not only survive but prosper. One must therefore assume that factors besides clinical competence exist that influence the referral decisions of PCPs.

Like patients do when choosing a PCP, primary care providers assume a certain acceptable level of competence among most specialists as the minimum ante for remaining on the medical staff of a local hospital (although there is the occasional outlier who has managed to stay in practice despite poor outcomes). The factors that actually distinguish these competent specialists from one another have little to do with clinical competence. In fact, changing PCP referral patterns in many communities can be as simple as introducing the specialist over dinner! This fact makes PCP referral retention a critical factor in any successful specialty practice that has competitors in the marketplace. Some unbelievers have been convinced the hard way as soon as a competent substitute moved to town.

Wise specialty physicians, those we want in our demand chain, understand the critical nature of the PCP relationship. They pay close attention to the needs, wants, and priorities of their PCP customers and establish the policies, procedures, and practice infrastructure needed to retain their referral relationships. Their efforts can be divided into three simple categories: access, respect, and always returning the patient.

Access

When a PCP decides to refer a patient for specialty care, the dynamics of the primary care encounter change. Most patients are not prepared to select their own specialist; they rely totally on their PCP for a recommendation. Thus, the PCP is in the wonderful position of being able to direct referrals as he sees fit. However, the PCP's patient relationship is then at risk. If the specialist fails to perform in terms of clinical quality of care or caring, the PCP will probably hear about it. Given the patient's likely anxiety level, access becomes a key factor in meeting the patient's priorities and, if the potential condition is serious, the PCP's priorities too.

Access as it relates to a specialty practice involves time, timeliness, and payer participation. Wise specialists are willing to make themselves available to communicate with their referring physicians regarding particular cases or questions both before and after the specialty visit. They are also willing to see the referred patient in a timely manner to relieve patient anxiety or to meet the desires of a concerned PCP. Successful specialists realize that their payer participation will likely mirror that of their primary care referral sources. The wise specialist will gladly see the Medicaid or self-pay patient as readily as the well-insured patient to meet not only the patient's clinical needs but also the PCP's needs. No wise specialist will turn away a request from a PCP because of a patient's method of payment, creating embarrassment for the PCP in the process.

Invasive specialty physicians must balance their schedule to allow adequate time for patient evaluation and follow-up as well as procedures. This balancing act presents a real challenge for busy practices, especially if operating rooms or procedure rooms are difficult to schedule. Some specialists have successfully brought nurse practitioners or physician assistants into their practices to increase their efficiency during procedures and to provide evaluation and management services. These well-trained extenders can leverage the physician's time while providing or facilitating excellent and timely care for patients and responsiveness to PCPs. Other specialists have invested in their own ambulatory procedure rooms and surgical centers in search of greater practice flexibility. Some busy specialists wisely engage their primary care referral sources in postprocedure management activities, which, if managed correctly, increase the referral tie to the PCP and deepen the relationship. (This issue is discussed in more detail later in the chapter.)

Respect (On Their Terms)

In addition to providing patient access, the successful specialist possesses and demonstrates respect for PCPs. The specialist ensures that this respect is reflected in every aspect of her office or surgical practice. Too often specialists express their superior knowledge or skill in a relatively narrow field through intolerance or even contempt for PCPs whom they perceive to have less skill, training, or experience. Rather than viewing PCPs as customers and partners in the delivery of quality healthcare, pompous specialists spend more time viewing themselves and their tools as the be-all and end-all for patients lucky enough to come within their grasp. Fortunately for their patients, the majority of these "technicians" are skilled and do meet their clinical needs. But they have little respect for anyone but themselves, doing little to contribute to the quality of healthcare outside of their own small sphere. Frustrated PCPs see these types of specialists as high-paid technicians and use them begrudgingly until a competent alternative becomes available.

Contrast these technicians with successful specialists who demonstrate respect for and build a partnership with PCPs for the benefit of the community. That respect is demonstrated in several ways, as follows.

Knowing the Referral Sources

Intuitively or otherwise, successful specialists understand and value the role of PCPs as the "relationship providers" in the complex world of medicine. They understand that Mrs. Smith and her family rely on that PCP to provide preventive services and to provide (or provide access to) more invasive services during times of illness or injury. Successful specialists understand that they are dependent on these PCPs for their bread and butter. They understand who their referral sources are and they pay attention to the number of referrals they receive from each source each month.

Providing Access

Successful specialists understand the critical and delicate nature of patient referrals, particularly in competitive markets, where PCPs have a choice of competent physicians in each specialty. Consequently, they take the time to provide consults, they assess referred patients in a timely manner, and they participate with the payers used by their primary care partners, sometimes even to their own financial detriment.

Acknowledging Referrals

Through personal phone conversations, postoperative written communication, interaction in the medical staff lounge, and other means, successful specialists acknowledge and thank PCPs for their referrals. They also use such occasions to solicit feedback from these critical customers regarding the PCP's needs, wants, and priorities in the relationship.

Engaging PCPs

The wisest (and often busiest) specialists engage their primary care referral sources in the diagnosis and treatment of their referred patients. Granted that some PCPs are not interested in following these cases because of their own busy schedules, but many relish the opportunity to remain connected, particularly with intriguing and complex medical challenges. Taking a few moments to discuss the case with the PCP, either during or after the examination, and confirming or enhancing the PCP's diagnosis have the dual benefit of cementing the relationship and improving the PCP's ability to diagnose other cases in the future. Engaging the PCP in a discussion of the proposed treatment plan has the same effect and sets up the opportunity for coordinated follow-up by the PCP (remember that old "coordination of care" concept?).

Complimenting Decisions

I purchased a new vehicle some time ago and talked with my mechanic about eventually putting 200,000 miles on it. He responded favorably, indicating that I had chosen the right brand to achieve such a goal. (Of course, he is also willing to help me keep the vehicle in shape during those 200,000 miles.) His comment was a compliment, not only to the manufacturer of the brand but also to me as the wise purchaser of such a vehicle. His sincere compliment also strengthened my relationship with him. We all like to be told we have made good choices. Successful specialists understand that medical retail customers are no different. They want to know they have made a good choice in selecting a PCP. Pausing to offer a sincere compliment to the patient regarding the PCP does not detract from, but rather enhances, the specialist's standing in the patient's mind. Of course, some of these compliments will surely reach the PCP and further cement the professional relationship.

Never Denigrating

One of the most disheartening messages a specialist can deliver to a patient, either directly or indirectly, is that the PCP misdiagnosed an ailment. When the PCP and the specialist disagree (or when specialists disagree among themselves), the patient's confidence is shaken. Here, the patient is like a child who has watched mom and dad argue and is left helpless and insecure, fearful of the potential outcome. Wise specialists never "fight in front of the kids." There may be those occasions when the only affirming remark a specialist can make to the patient involves the wisdom of the PCP in sending the patient for further evaluation. For the benefit of the patient, to maintain the relationship, and to educate the PCP, wise specialists never denigrate the PCP, especially in front of the patient. Instead, they discuss the diagnosis with the PCP in private and work with the physician to develop a treatment plan. This process ensures high-quality care, educates the PCP regarding future similar situations and patients, and maintains the professional relationship.

Sharing Knowledge

Specialists have usually developed both technical skills and cognitive knowledge of certain disease states or conditions. Through extra personal effort and experience they have prepared themselves to offer services that are unique and specialized. But a few foolish specialists may assume that their unique skills and knowledge entitle them to stand above other physicians on a medical staff and to remain aloof. Such an attitude damages the reputation of the specialist and overlooks the tremendous community good that comes from sharing knowledge. A majority of the specialists with whom we have worked believe that sharing their specialized knowledge is an obligation that accrues to the benefit of the profession. The most successful specialists, in fact, make such sharing a continual part of their practice. They have a propensity to teach. They use formal educational forums, patient feedback to PCPs, telephone consults, and a variety of other methods to share their knowledge in a manner that is appropriate and not overbearing. These specialists recognize the value of enhancing the diagnostic and therapeutic skills of their PCP peers in the specialist's particular area of expertise.

Testing Responsibly

Few actions insult a PCP and frustrate a patient more than a specialist reordering diagnostic tests already completed by the PCP. If such testing is warranted, and sometimes it is, the wise specialist will view this decision as an opportunity to engage the PCP. The patient will be informed that both physicians feel a need to reorder the diagnostic test and why.

Following Up

Successful specialists have learned what their primary care referring physicians prefer in terms of feedback and contact. They understand that different PCP personalities and practice levels require different forms of feedback and timing. How do they come to understand these preferences? They ask. Such relationship management can be informal (visits in the doctors' lounge or during medical staff meetings) or more formal (routine solicitation of feedback during telephone consults or through a brief survey).

Always Returning the Patient

The third and final rule for building strong relationships between the specialist and the PCP is to always return the patient. This sounds simple enough, but it can be quite challenging, particularly for nonsurgical internal medicine physicians who are treating chronic ailments as opposed to surgical cases. When given the opportunity, some patients prefer to have the specialist take over their primary care, and some PCPs prefer to have the specialist assume the referred patient's primary care. Other PCPs prefer to have the patient returned. Failure on the part of the specialist to understand the PCP's preference and to respond accordingly is likely to result in fewer future referrals. Once again, wise specialists understand this reality and consult with the PCP before making any commitments to the patient.

Some may think this stance is disingenuous on the part of the specialist, who may be perceived as putting her practice needs and the preferences of the PCP before those of the patient—and this is certainly a legitimate concern. However, no honorable PCP or specialist is going to place the patient's clinical needs in jeopardy. If the patient needs to remain in the care of the specialist for clinical reasons, that factor overrides all others, even if it means that the specialist risks losing a referral source. In addition, the specialist must reconcile the needs, wants, and priorities of both the individual patient and the referring physician or risk being unavailable (because of business failure) for future patients. Both the patient and the PCP are essential customers whose preferences must be carefully weighed, especially if they are in conflict. Honest dialog on the part of both physicians is critical in such situations. Such dialog is easier if the specialist has not cannibalized the PCP's practice in the past.

For the benefit of the demand chain, one cannot leave to chance the opportunity to find specialty physicians who understand or are willing to become the "specialist of choice" for referring physicians. One need only ask local PCPs to identify the specialty physicians they would include in a successful demand chain. Chapters 5 and 8 explore the role of the hospital, particularly the CEO, in strengthening the specialty ranks and managing this important component of the demand chain.

CHAPTER 5

The Role of the Hospital

This chapter presents five concepts:

- Your neighborhood gathering place
- The workshop
- Centers of excellence
- Community safety net
- Strategic integrator

This chapter explores why the hospital is the most appropriate place for integrating and fully developing the medical services demand chain. It examines the natural role of the hospital as a gathering place for medical staff members, many of whom still provide a large share of their services in and through the hospital; discusses the hospital as a "workshop" in the context of new competitive challenges; and examines the hospital's ability to combine medical expertise, technology, and marketing savvy to focus on individual service lines. The role of the full-service hospital as a safety net for the community is also discussed. Finally, the chapter looks at the role of the hospital as the strategic integrator of services, with the administrative staff, location, capital, and planning horizon necessary to travel the lengthy path toward developing a medical services demand chain.

CONCEPT 1: YOUR NEIGHBORHOOD GATHERING PLACE

We are fortunate to have a great family restaurant in our hometown. It is called Max & Erma's and the sign above the door says, "Your Neighborhood Gathering Place." And, indeed, Max & Erma's does seem to be the gathering place for people of all ages. Even the finicky high school crowd will frequently be found enjoying burgers, fries, pasta, or desserts after a local football game or performance. Adults can find more formal fare in delicious steaks, chicken, and fish, all consistently prepared and moderately priced. We frequently meet our close neighbors and distant friends to enjoy the food and relaxed atmosphere. You might say that Max & Erma's appears to have identified the needs, wants, and priorities of our neighborhood. The chain has effectively implemented a formula for success, which has been replicated in a variety of towns across the Midwest.

In most communities the hospital is a gathering place of sorts. By the nature of its position in the demand chain, the hospital has also been the "workshop" for all inpatient activities and, until recent years, all outpatient services too. Even in markets where the competitive landscape has been modified by specialty hospitals, ambulatory surgery centers, freestanding imaging centers, and the like, the hospital remains the common ground for most medical specialties. It is the place where PCPs admit their patients for inpatient services and follow them personally or through a hospitalist or intensivist. It is the place where most invasive diagnostic tests are performed. Most surgeries are performed within the hospital walls, particularly those that require the services of several specialties during the diagnosis, treatment, and recovery periods. The hospital is the place where physicians in several specialties gather to discuss a particularly perplexing intensive care patient. It is also the site where a variety of ancillary services are available to support inpatient and outpatient service delivery. Many of these services would not survive as stand-alone businesses, but as part of an integrated service they become essential components of a successful outcome. Most importantly, the hospital workshop provides patient beds to house those who are gravely ill, awaiting test results, preparing for procedures, or recovering from procedures.

Although the makeup of medical staffs has evolved over the years, the medical staff forum is still an integral part of the hospital as the "neighborhood gathering place." Most medical staffs are organized to credential physicians to admit patients and perform procedures within the hospital. Larger medical staffs are organized around departments to share best practices and improve the quality of patient care. They meet periodically to learn from one another, discussing mutual challenges and dealing with administrative matters such as scheduling emergency-department call coverage or hospital policies. The medical staff is a volunteer organization, and its members have varying levels of commitment, depending on their interests, their stage in life, their personalities, and the success of their own medical practices. Usually, a few leaders who are elected by their peers do a good share of the work. Often, the leadership positions are occupied only briefly—a blessing when the leader is inadequate, a curse when an excellent leader must move on. The vice president of medical affairs or hospital support staff performs much of the administrative work associated with the medical staff.

Today the relationships between hospitals and their volunteer medical staffs are strained by conflicting objectives and interests. Many diagnostic tests and therapeutic procedures formerly requiring hospitalization or hospital capital now are performed in medical offices. Physician-owned ambulatory surgery centers have appeared in many communities, siphoning precious surgical cases (usually well-insured cases) away from hospitals. These realities make it much more difficult for hospital executives to have meaningful strategic discussions with medical staff members when some of them compete with the hospital for prime business. Despite the challenges of this volunteer body, however, no other forum outside the hospital setting can gather physicians for the benefit of the hospital and the communities served.

CONCEPT 2: THE WORKSHOP

Many of today's hospitals have a rich history dating back several decades. Some of the oldest hospitals can trace their history to the mid-nineteenth century, when they were founded and sponsored by religious orders after the Civil War. These early hospitals provided two essential services that remain vital today. First, they served as a place where the sick and injured could recover under the watchful care of nurses. Second, they provided a "workshop" for physicians who previously practiced their trade in small offices or in their patients' homes. Medical professionals at the time had few tools and even fewer medications to support their relatively limited knowledge. In fact, they provided more caring than actual clinical care.

Today's medical technology, knowledge, and medications exceed even the wildest dreams of physicians and nurses serving just a few decades ago. However, the fundamental role of the hospital has not changed. Hospitals provide a place where the sick and injured can rest and recover under the watchful eye of caring nursing staff. They also provide a workshop for physicians to diagnose and treat many ailments.

Other workshops have appeared, including freestanding ambulatory surgery centers and imaging centers. Improvements in technology have significantly increased the number of diagnostic and therapeutic procedures that can be performed in a medical office. However, when a patient is seriously ill or injured, the hospital is still the facility of choice for patients and providers alike.

From small rural facilities to large tertiary and quaternary medical centers, the anatomy of a hospital workshop is amazing. Consider the emergency department alone. Open 24 hours a day, 365 days a year, its physicians, nurses, technicians, and clerks serve

20 to 30 patients each day in smaller hospitals and upwards of 200 patients each day in the largest facilities. The emergency department must be equipped and prepared to diagnose and provide immediate treatment for the simplest of ailments as well as for the complex cases that inspire top-rated television dramas. Positioned at the "bottom of the cliff," emergency departments must be prepared to deal with the trauma and tragedies we hear about on the morning news and read about in the newspaper. Emergency departments are the workshops where the ill and injured have access to the equipment and skilled professionals who can stabilize, diagnose, and treat myriad emergent and nonemergent events. There is no other place like it. There is no substitute for it.

In addition, every real hospital has labor-and-delivery rooms and an associated nursery. From small, relatively unsophisticated rural facilities to large, urban women's centers with neonatal nurseries, hospitals are the birthing center of choice for most women and the workshop of choice for most obstetricians. The hospital obstetrics department brings together the facility, equipment, nursing staff, anesthesiologists, and pediatricians necessary to support Mrs. Smith and her physician during a normal vaginal birth. The department is linked to operating rooms for Cesarean sections, and it also stabilizes and supports the newborn, whether the baby is normal and healthy or requires continued life support outside the womb. Again, there is no other place like it and no substitute for it.

Now consider the intensive care unit (ICU) or critical care unit of a hospital. The ICU's combination of technology, facilities, and professional skill tips the balance between life and death. This corner of the hospital is where the sickest and the most severely injured patients are found. The family and friends of ICU patients gather in waiting rooms where the anxiety is often palpable. In this setting, medical professionals are engaged in some of life's most significant dramas. The ICU routinely tests the skills of the most highly trained medical professionals as they deal with multisystem failures, severe trauma, and death. Battles that would have been lost just a few years ago are won today through new and powerful drugs that are carefully administered and balanced, while technology keeps ailing patients breathing and monitors their vital signs. Some medical professionals become callous to the intensive care drama, perhaps to protect their own emotions and decision-making skills. Others, however, seem to have the capacity for endless compassion, extending their medical skill not only to the patient but also to the patient's family. Regardless, the hospital ICU is one of a kind. There is no competition trying to steal away the cream and no substitute for this stage on which life and death and an occasional miracle are played out.

Of course, these high-profile departments could not survive without the many mundane but essential supporting departments. Think of a hospital without a laboratory. How about radiology? Think of the rehabilitation departments where patients often make progress at a snail's pace. Consider the complexities of keeping the hospital clean and sanitary or of maintaining its numerous physical plant systems and subsystems. The administrative departments (sometimes viewed by physicians as necessary evils) are essential to the continued viability and growth of the workshop. The hospital may even be a morgue for those who have lost the battle for life. And last but not least, where would we be if we could not criticize the food services department?

Despite the small percentage of clinical or service quality aberrations, despite the challenges from ambulatory surgery centers and diagnostic centers, despite poor reimbursement for some services, and despite myriad other challenges, there is no place like and no substitute for a full-service community hospital.

CONCEPT 3: CENTERS OF EXCELLENCE

Centers of excellence emerged in more aggressive markets in the 1980s. They were the hospital industry's equivalent of a product-line or service-line organization—a management approach commonly used in other industries to improve the quality of products and services as well as the responsiveness to customers. Common hospital service lines include women's services, cardiac care, cancer care, behavioral medicine, and orthopedics.

Centers of excellence often combine the latest in technology, physicians with unique skills, specially trained support staff, a specialized physical plant, and consumer marketing in an attempt to create a superior level of clinical and service quality that will differentiate the service line and the hospital from competitors. Being known as "the heart hospital" or "the premier cancer center" seems to have a halo effect, enhancing the public's perception of the hospital's entire portfolio of service offerings.

Successful service lines have indeed contributed in several ways to the quality of clinical services and to service delivery. This contribution is a result of several factors, as follows.

Volume

The old adage "practice makes perfect" is certainly relevant to service lines. It stands to reason (and is generally accepted among healthcare professionals) that a busier program promotes a better clinical outcome. A hospital with a high annual volume of coronary artery bypass grafting procedures is likely to have patients who experience fewer complications (and more effective management of those that do occur) than a hospital where fewer such procedures are performed, because the high-volume team is experienced in preoperative, surgical, and postoperative care.

Innovation

Innovation occurs more frequently in service-line settings where expertise is developed both individually and by service delivery teams. Volume provides experience and routine, fostering incremental improvement in processes and efficiencies in the delivery of clinical care. Such improvement may not be documented in medical journals, but it is clearly resident as intellectual and technical capital in physicians, technicians, and nursing staff.

Technology

Successful service lines generate the ability to achieve a financial return, which attracts capital for new technology to further enhance the service line. The newest and latest equipment often supports innovation and improved outcomes. An organization striving to achieve a distinctive competence in a particular service line is likely to find, acquire, and use the latest equipment to support that effort.

Focus

As with product-line strategies in other industries, hospital service lines tend to focus the attention of clinicians and management on better understanding and meeting not only the clinical needs of patients but also the needs, wants, and priorities of targeted customers. Maternity care is perhaps the most common example, often bringing together clinical expertise and technology in a room that looks more like a five-star hotel and spa than a delivery room. Several obstetricians with whom I have worked indicate that many of their patients "shop" the labor-and-delivery rooms of local hospitals to select which facility they like best—a rather unusual phenomenon in most patient–hospital interactions.

In the early days of service lines, competition was relatively genteel. One facility became the heart hospital. Another invested in radiation therapy. A third developed expertise in orthopedics. By the early 1990s such mild competition was long gone in many markets. Money and a positive image in the community tended to follow expertise in cardiac care. Hospitals with enough financial resources moved quickly to establish open-heart surgery programs and then to build an army of cardiologists as less-invasive techniques became available. Cath labs made state-of-the-art cardiac care available to hospitals even without open-heart programs. More recently, physicians have teamed up with for-profit companies to build their own specialty heart hospitals in several communities, making it even more difficult to achieve a unique reputation in the provision of cardiac care. Cancer care has followed a similar route, with groups of oncologists now offering sophisticated care in their own specialized facilities outside the traditional hospital campus.

Competition is intense for these and similar service lines in many communities. The achievement of a sustainable competitive advantage under such circumstances is difficult at best, and the attempt to compete can be financially disastrous. I watched one organization pour millions of dollars into a new heart hospital in a large metropolitan area that already had more than a dozen open-heart programs, including an investor-owned specialty heart hospital. The result was a beautiful facility that lost millions of dollars each month as it tried to cannibalize several existing programs, including its own sister facilities in the same community.

CONCEPT 4: COMMUNITY SAFETY NET

By the 1950s, religiously sponsored hospitals were common in many communities around the United States. Most of these organizations have traditionally served the needs of those who presented at their doors, regardless of these patients' ability to pay. In fact, in many states the charitable mission of most hospitals has been acknowledged with the abatement of taxes on their income. The tax-exempt status of many hospitals continues today.

Despite the legal challenges leveled at many not-for-profit hospitals for their alleged aggressive pricing and collection techniques, they have traditionally been the safety net for the poor and underserved in communities throughout the United States. While the number of underinsured and uninsured Americans makes great political fodder for campaign speeches, while access remains a major problem, and while debates over community health and socialized medicine rage on, hospitals are still treating patients who present with emergent conditions, regardless of their ability to pay. They also continue to serve patients covered only by federal and state government programs, despite the huge write-offs that apply. Bad debt write-offs and contractual write-offs have a substantial impact on the financial statements of all community hospitals.

Often forgotten or not considered at all is the fact that some services offered by community hospitals could not survive as stand-alone businesses, including some maternity services and emergency departments. Many for-profit companies in other industries would not long tolerate such financially marginal service lines. Hospitals in many communities also provide education and disease screening to enhance awareness and promote health in the communities they serve.

A complex set of interactions between various service lines and payment sources allows hospitals to continue seeing the uninsured and underinsured while still amassing enough capital to service debt and remain competitive. Hospitals are often criticized for cost-shifting from payers with purchasing power to payers and individuals with less negotiating leverage, rather than being as charitable as they should be to warrant their tax-exempt status. I certainly cannot argue against the reality that some payers and individuals bear a larger burden than others, nor would I attempt to justify the huge salaries paid to some hospital and health system executives or to senior executives in other industries. I can only relate my experience with several hospitals and clinics that were struggling to serve the underserved and writing off hundreds of thousands of dollars annually as bad debt—legitimate charity care to patients who lack the ability (and sometimes the desire) to pay, regardless of the pricing strategy involved. I have attended meetings and participated in discussions in which decisions were made to lose $250,000, $500,000, or $1 million a year on certain service lines or community health projects to maintain access for patients who need the services and cannot find them elsewhere. I have raised my hand to approve the charity care policies that are put in place to assist those with legitimate needs and circumstances.

Even though hospital administration today is largely in the hands of lay management professionals, the hospital-sponsoring bodies often maintain some influence on boards of trustees or have a representative mission officer to ensure that management considers the needs of the underserved. These officers frequently have tremendous influence on the discernment and decisions of the lay administrators who are the board-appointed fiduciaries. The mission-based perspective in many hospitals and health systems is alive and well, although it must continually be balanced with the realities of staying in business to continue providing a safety net to the communities they serve.

CONCEPT 5: STRATEGIC INTEGRATOR

Although integration has fallen on hard times in the healthcare arena, it is nonetheless critical to a competitive demand-chain strategy. Imagine a hospital and its medical staff having a common focus, uniting to implement a retail strategy by placing affiliated PCPs within a ten-minute drive of every urban and suburban home within the combined hospital–medical staff geographic market. Imagine that this partnership is also establishing rural clinic sites in viable secondary markets. Imagine the proper mix of qualified specialists who understand the retail customer and the PCP customer and who organize to meet their respective needs, wants, and priorities. Imagine a hospital that provides services of outstanding quality and caters to the needs, wants, and priorities of its physicians and retail customers. Think of hospital-based specialists, including anesthesiologists, radiologists, pathologists, and hospitalists, whose clinical skills and customer service are second to none. Imagine these demand-chain members all cooperatively focused on meeting Mrs. Smith's needs, wants, and priorities.

Contrast this integrated demand chain with the more traditional nonintegrated set of medical services found in most communities. Relationships between specialists and PCPs are left to chance. The hospital CEO thinks her job is to keep the surgeons happy and to run an efficient workshop. Precious little communication occurs among the parties and with PCPs. In fact, the hospital CEO has not even met many of the PCPs who use or refer to the specialists who use the hospital! As amazing as this may sound, some hospital CEOs have never even met some of the PCPs that are employed by the hospital, let alone those who are independent. Neither the CEO nor the hospital management team knows where the PCPs are referring patients for services or whether the PCPs are satisfied with the available specialists. The loudest physicians on the medical staff usually identify performance problems with the workshop, while the concerns of the majority go unheard and unaddressed.

Which of these two demand chains will win the competitive battle? Which one will provide consistently superior, coordinated clinical care? Which one will ensure that every patient/customer has a positive experience, regardless of access point or duration? Which demand chain will attract and retain high-quality specialists because of a guaranteed flow of referrals? Which one will attract and retain a large cadre of PCPs who feel valued by the specialists and the affiliated hospital(s)? Which demand chain will ultimately lose market share?

Leading firms in multiple industries have demonstrated the competitive power and effectiveness of successful integration. (Both vertical and horizontal integration have long been considered viable approaches in many competitive settings.) The ability to organize and focus all demand-chain members on the needs, wants, and priorities of the end user—the retail customer—is considered a phenomenal potential strategic advantage. In *From Mind to Market—Reinventing the Retail Supply Chain*,

Roger Blackwell (1997) identifies several leading firms that have used integration strategies successfully. These firms include retailer Wal-Mart, distributor Nike, and wholesaler Cardinal Health. Blackwell also notes that different firms use different approaches to achieve their integration objectives. Some rely on ownership of various demand-chain components, while others use strategic partnerships and other collaborative approaches. Factors such as size, capital, market position, competitive dominance, customer access, and management capabilities can influence the ability of any one of the demand-chain members to serve as the strategic integrator for all of the other components.

Given the self-interest, the time and energy, the access to capital, the medical staff infrastructure, and the planning horizon found among the various medical services demand-chain members, the hospital is in the best position to serve as the integrator of medical services along the demand chain. Identifying the hospital as the most likely demand-chain integrator will probably raise eyebrows and ire in some circles. Certainly, some vie to occupy such a position, but their arguments in most markets are hollow. Consider the following.

Self-Interest

The hospital (and by extension, the hospital-based physician specialists) has a strong incentive to make the demand chain work to ensure its own survival. The medical staff is the most common manifestation of this incentive. Through both formal and informal medical staff development (a critical component of demand-chain management), hospital executives routinely attempt to identify and attract the specialists needed to sustain the hospital's basic services and service lines. Many physicians, by comparison, are not dependent on a particular hospital for the success of their medical practices. They can (and many do) conduct their business at multiple facilities in their communities.

Time and Energy

Hospitals often employ or have access to the financial, legal, planning, marketing, and other administrative expertise and infrastructure that can focus time and energy on integration strategies. Physicians, on the other hand, are usually the chief source of production in their offices and spend a majority of their time focused on the clinical needs of their patients and the preferences of their referring physicians. Administrative duties of any kind are usually dealt with after hours at the expense of personal and family time. Some physicians have joined "the dark side" (as some may joke) by becoming full-time administrators. Most are found working for hospitals, because medical clinics cannot afford or will not fund non-producing, high-salary human resources.

Gathering Place

The hospital workshop provides a physical gathering place for many physicians, and the medical staff infrastructure is a natural forum for discussing issues, ideas, personal agendas, and concerns. (Granted, many formal medical staffs are struggling to remain relevant in today's highly competitive markets, but most are still a potentially significant force.) No other vehicle can compete with the power of an effective medical staff organization to drive the demand chain in partnership with management.

Capital Development

Despite reimbursement challenges, uncompensated care, specialty hospitals, ambulatory surgery centers, not-for-profit litigation, and other threats, hospitals are still in the best position of any demand-chain member to accumulate capital. Physicians, particularly multispecialty groups, have or can obtain the intellectual talent and provide the gathering place needed to drive the integration process. A few integrated practices, such as the Mayo Clinic and the Cleveland Clinic, have demonstrated that they can generate capital. However, the majority of medical practices in most communities, even larger multispecialty groups, lack the discipline to fund their own depreciation, let alone amass capital.

Planning Horizon

Finally, the nature of the hospital business lends itself to a longer planning horizon than that found in most medical practices. The goal of most small medical group practices is to pay the bills and maximize short-term income for the physician shareholders. Given limited administrative time and limited capital, physician group leaders focus their energies on initiatives that will produce the greatest short-term return. Hospital executives, on the other hand, must (or are supposed to) answer to boards of trustees/directors, sponsors, and shareholders for both short-term and long-term performance.

In short, hospitals have the self-interest, staff with time and energy, capacity to serve as a gathering place, access to capital, and lengthy planning horizon necessary to fully develop a medical services demand chain. Based on the strength of their leadership, hospitals are in the best position to serve as integrators of all the demand-chain members.

REFERENCE

Blackwell, R. D. 1997. *From Mind to Market—Reinventing the Retail Supply Chain.* New York: HarperCollins.

CHAPTER 6

The Role of Hospital-Based Physicians

This chapter presents three concepts:

- Hospital-based physicians as retailers
- Hospital-based specialists as providers of choice
- Hospital-based specialists as hospital partners

Each year my associates and I interview hundreds of physicians, most of whom are PCPs. During the interviews we often learn a great deal about the hospital or hospitals they use and the specialty physicians associated with those hospitals. During one such interview, a family practice physician who happened to be employed by our hospital client discussed the barriers to his use of hospital services. Like several of his peers, he reported frustration with the group of radiologists with whom the hospital contracted to provide its imaging services. The radiology group had developed a reputation for being inflexible in patient scheduling, which resulted in long delays for some imaging procedures, and the radiologists were perceived as not being responsive to the referring physicians' inquiries and requests. The family practitioner noted that scheduling a patient for a mammogram often resulted in a four-week wait, whereas the competing hospital and radiology group could see a patient within a week. He noted that the competitor's radiology group always acted like they welcomed and wanted his business.

Just imagine the consequences of this scenario being repeated several times each year in the practices of employed and independent primary and specialty care providers. The financial implications are significant, as are the risks of sending market share on a golden platter into the hands of a competitor.

On another occasion, I interviewed an anesthesiologist who was employed by a hospital. He expressed frustration with a large independent group of anesthesiologists who refused to schedule their time for afternoon surgical cases more than 24 hours in advance, creating scheduling frustrations for busy surgeons, their patients, and the hospital. No amount of pleading or cajoling could convince these critical specialists to change their pattern of "potential afternoons off."

In another market, several primary care and specialty physicians openly shared their enthusiasm for a recently contracted group of emergency physicians who had taken over the hospital's emergency department. Frequent patient complaints of tortuous three-hour emergency department waits had been replaced with a widely communicated guarantee that all patients would be seen by an emergency physician within 30 minutes of their arrival and would be discharged or admitted for further treatment within 90 minutes.

The success of this initiative was infectious, as multiple departments stepped up to the plate to make the guarantee become a reality. Even independent physicians reportedly were more enthusiastic about taking emergency department calls. Such success breeds additional performance improvement initiatives. Everyone wants to be on the winning side.

Hospital-based physicians have a unique and challenging role in the medical services demand chain. They support a variety of hospital departments and service lines. They are a critical component of many invasive tests and procedures. To be successful they must meet the varied needs, wants, and priorities of at least three major customer segments. They must be prepared to have direct contact with patients and their family members, often under adverse circumstances.

They must be the providers of choice for referring physicians. They must be effective partners to physicians who use the hospital and its departments as their workshop.

Hospital-based specialties commonly include anesthesiology, radiology, pathology, hospitalist, and the emergency department.

CONCEPT 1: HOSPITAL-BASED PHYSICIANS AS RETAILERS

The emergency department is a world all its own. It is one of the few hospital departments to which a patient can self-refer. Many patients do so for truly emergent situations, but others do so because they do not have a traditional primary care relationship. Very few community hospitals or tertiary referral centers escape the negative lore associated with emergency departments. Stories of insufferable emergency department waits and bleeding limbs abound and are held in sharp contrast to situations portrayed on television shows. Of course, few of these extremes actually represent reality, but the customer's perception is reality.

Suburban hospital emergency departments reflect the demographics of their surroundings, treating well-insured patients and a variety of common injuries and illnesses. The emergency department is a tremendous source of patients for the suburban hospital and its affiliated specialists. Urban hospital executives, on the other hand, might view their emergency departments as a necessary evil. Large, urban emergency departments often reflect the consequences of poverty, inadequate health insurance, and lack of access to proper physical and mental healthcare. Inner-city locations often represent the ugly side of society—the portion that the rest of us choose to ignore. Armed security guards and city police help clinicians cope with the true costs of poverty, drugs, crime, and a variety of social ills. Emergency doctors in some inner-city hospitals find it difficult to identify community physicians, either specialists or PCPs, who are willing to accept unattached patients.

Regardless of the location, for the patient whose pain is reduced, whose injury is stabilized, whose illness is treated, or whose life is saved, the emergency department is a miraculous blessing. Add to this medical miracle a caring culture, a "fast track" for nonemergent situations, pleasant surroundings, and even a performance guarantee, and the hospital emergency department is a phenomenal access point for patients and their families.

A retail component of the practices is associated with other hospital-based physicians. For example, anesthesiologists have precious little time to establish any rapport with their patients and often encounter patients and their families at the most anxious of times, shortly before surgery or childbirth. Pathologists rarely see the patient/customer, but their influence and customer service attitude are often present in phlebotomists, who may serve hundreds of customers each day. Likewise, radiologists providing diagnostic services are often shielded from direct contact with patients, but their attitudes, schedules, clinical performance, and personal productivity directly affect the ability of the hospital, radiation technologists, and support staff to meet patient needs, wants, and priorities.

CONCEPT 2: HOSPITAL-BASED SPECIALISTS AS PROVIDERS OF CHOICE

Hospitalist programs have taken hold in many communities around the country but rarely without some angst on the part of PCPs, who are accustomed to following their own patients. The ability to win the hearts of PCPs and attract their business appears to be a function of several factors. Hospitalists who have been most successful at facilitating the transition have the following characteristics:

- *Accessibility.* The group must have enough physicians to provide around-the-clock coverage 365 days a year to be able to attract patient referrals from community physicians.

- *Stability.* Having the same face(s) and name(s) over time is essential for building trust with PCPs and with other specialty physicians.
- *Clinical competence.* Demonstrating clinical competence and confidence, especially at critical times, requires a team of hospitalists who are A-players—no exceptions!
- *Responsiveness.* Hospitalists who have the ability to communicate often and well with referring physicians, admitting physicians, consulting physicians, hospital support staff, and patients are likely to have far greater success than those who are clinically competent but lack communication skills.
- *Productivity.* Hospitalists who possess the ability to effectively and efficiently see a large volume of patients and to "flex" with admission volume breed confidence among support staff members, ancillary services providers, and others.
- *Retail customer service.* A hospitalist may be accountable for coordinating the services of several other members of the demand chain who are focused on the patient/customer. A hospitalist's ability to understand not just the clinical needs but also the personal needs, wants, and priorities of the patient and her "chaperones" is a critical component of successful implementation. In addition, the hospitalist most often is the face of the demand chain for patients and their family members during a hospital stay, a time when the patient is most ill and may feel insecure and vulnerable.

The successful hospitalist group becomes a phenomenal integrator and coordinator of services and care, partnering with several experts and support personnel to achieve the desired outcome for all concerned.

The hospitalist becomes an extension of the primary care physician in the hospital setting. He is available 24/7, is an expert at hospital care, and becomes adept at marshalling hospital resources to meet the patient's needs. The hospitalist communicates effectively with other specialists involved in the efficient coordination of services. Most importantly, wise hospitalists never forget that they are treating Dr. Smith's or Dr. Jones's patient, and they respond to, communicate with, and engage these referring physicians according to each one's preference. The most effective hospitalists become partners with their referring physicians. They become, in effect, "the partner who has hospital call this week."

The need for partnership between anesthesiologists and surgeons is clear. Neither can work in the surgical suite without the other. Whether anesthesia is provided by a physician or a certified registered nurse anesthetist who is supervised by an anesthesiologist, the clinical, service, and emotional competence of the provider is on display at all times. The anesthesiologist must not only respond to the needs of the patient, she must also outshine the competition in meeting the surgeon's unique needs, wants, and priorities. Otherwise, the surgeon (particularly if she is among the best) will go elsewhere. Certain surgeons are definitely more difficult than others. Some surgeons have more natural talent and are more competent than others. Regardless, the wise anesthesiologist not only will meet the clinical requirements of each case but also will consciously build and improve the partnership with the surgeon for each case.

CONCEPT 3: HOSPITAL-BASED SPECIALISTS AS HOSPITAL PARTNERS

Hospital radiology and laboratory departments include a variety of technical and support personnel. The members of these departments often use sophisticated equipment to produce the diagnostic results critical to effective diagnosis and treatment of patients. However, neither department can function successfully without the clinical expertise of a physician, and neither department can function effectively without clinical leadership that understands and insists on excellence in customer service to patients, hospital support staff, and referring physicians (both primary and specialty care).

Consequently, to provide excellent clinical quality and service, hospitals must engage radiologists and pathologists who are more than competent clinicians. Even flawless technicians will fail if they cannot back up their clinical competence with service-quality leadership in partnership with the hospital and its staff members.

The best hospital partnerships have a fairly predictable set of characteristics, including the following.

Mutual Purpose

A shared vision, a common purpose, a joint venture, or a shared strategy: Regardless of the term and tactics used, the implication of this concept is the same. The foundation of successful physician–hospital partnerships is mutual purpose. That purpose is based on, but goes well beyond, providing quality clinical care. It incorporates not only mission, vision, and direction but also methods—tactics as well as strategies. Hospital-based physicians are in a unique position to partner with hospitals around a mutual purpose, particularly if the hospital is their only workshop. That mutual purpose must include the following:

- *Clinical quality.* Quality clinical care and outcomes drive mutual purpose in a healthcare setting. Appropriately meeting clinical needs is fundamental to our "reason for being."
- *Service quality.* Excellent service for all demand-chain members and their customers—patients, families, and referral sources—is essential to a sustained presence in increasingly competitive markets.
- *Financial viability.* Any mutual purpose must include mutual benefit. Otherwise, partners find themselves focused on Maslow's security and safety needs (i.e., in survival mode) rather

than on a higher purpose (Certo 1997). Financial viability for the hospital(s) and the physicians is essential and must be included in the mutual purpose.

- *Sustainability.* Any mutual purpose must be developed and tested against constantly changing industry and competitive trends. The endurance of a defined purpose is inextricably linked to its believability and the partnership's ability to attract and retain partners.

- *Compelling.* No purpose will truly be shared or enduring unless it is compelling for all parties involved. The mutual purpose cannot just support the hospital's mission, although that mission must be furthered. It cannot just address the physicians' agendas, although they must be genuinely addressed and not mentioned just to appease. A compelling purpose may be as simple as an emergency department guarantee or service-line superiority, or it may be as complex as meeting community need. Regardless, it must motivate behavior (usually behavior change), or it is not a mutual purpose.

Mutual Respect

Successful physician–hospital relationships thrive only in an environment and culture of mutual respect. That environment starts with a relationship-competent hospital CEO and effective physician leaders (usually medical staff leaders). In a culture of mutual respect, both physician and hospital leaders recognize and internalize the fact that to achieve their full potential they need the skills, abilities, perspectives, competence, and involvement of the other party. (Yes, I say "full potential" even in an environment of freestanding diagnostic imaging centers and ambulatory surgery centers!) In the absence of mutual respect, the statement of purpose written at a planning retreat will endure only long enough to be printed, framed, and hung on the wall as decoration. The only solution to lack of mutual respect may be to change the players at the table, starting with the hospital CEO.

Dialog

Several authors have discussed the concept of dialog leading to mutual understanding, mutual purpose, and mutual respect (Patterson et al. 2002; Porter 1998). Successful physician–hospital partnerships are nourished by true dialog—that is, the ability not only to identify the vision, purpose, or direction but also to agree on the right methods to achieve that purpose. It involves conversing under circumstances in which the parties disagree (sometimes strongly) or feel threatened and coming to the best solution to achieve the stated purpose. Dialog is the ability to question current methods in the face of performance facts or to respond to a compelling argument without becoming entrenched in and blinded by the status quo. It involves the ability to be honest in sharing opinions, experiences, and facts while simultaneously being respectful of the opinions, experiences, and facts presented by others. Its purpose is to identify *what* is right rather than who is right.

Accountability

Clear performance expectations, rigorous performance measurement, objective review, and commitment to endure the pain of performance improvement are all essential to achieving a true partnership between physicians and hospitals. (Accountability is discussed further in Chapter 11.)

Radiologists, pathologists, hospitalists, anesthesiologists, and other hospital-based physicians must develop a true partnership with hospital leadership based on the above principles if either party is to achieve its potential. Thankfully, these physicians are in a unique position to create just such a partnership with the right hospital and department or service-line leaders. The greatest challenge to such a partnership is the plethora of competitive alternatives for hospital-based physicians, such as splitting time at other acute care hospitals or ownership in competing limited-services facilities.

The essential role of hospital-based specialists in the demand chain is clear. Like other members of the demand chain, they are retailers who meet Mrs. Smith's needs, wants, and priorities either directly or through competent technicians. In addition, hospital-based specialists are in a unique position to partner with other specialists and with the hospital in meeting the needs, wants, and priorities of patients, their families, and other demand-chain members.

REFERENCES

Certo, S. C. 1997. *Supervision: Quality, Diversity, and Technology, 2nd ed.* New York: McGraw-Hill.

Patterson, K., J. Grenny, R. McMillan, and A. Switzler. 2002. *Crucial Conversations: Tools for Talking When Stakes Are High.* New York: McGraw-Hill.

Porter, M. E. 1998. *Competitive Advantage: Creating and Sustaining Superior Performance.* New York: The Free Press.

CHAPTER 7

Developing and Implementing a Retail Strategy

This chapter presents three concepts:

- Our fundamental mission
- The process of retail analysis
- Retail implementation tactics

As I mentioned in the Introduction, this book will be of interest to senior hospital and health system executives. This chapter will be of particular interest to those who are charged with the responsibility for increasing their hospital's market share. (It will also be valuable for multispecialty group strategists.) My colleagues and I frequently work with senior teams to analyze who holds the market share in their primary and secondary markets (as defined by zip codes) that produces the majority of their throughput (admissions). Our analysis also identifies areas of market-share vulnerability because of poor primary care coverage or competitor incursions/dominance in certain geographic areas. Armed with this information and data on population trends, migration patterns, and retail corridors, hospital executives are in a good position to develop and implement tactics that can lock in their market share for years to come. This chapter details the process that I call "retail analysis and strategy development."

CONCEPT 1: OUR FUNDAMENTAL MISSION

Previous chapters described the medical services demand chain and the roles of each stakeholder—the customer, the PCP, the specialist, the hospital, and the hospital-based specialist—in the success or failure of that chain. We now shift our focus to the process of implementing a medical services demand chain, beginning with the fundamental mission to capture (or, as Drucker says, "create") customers. In general, customers determine which organizations (healthcare or otherwise) ultimately survive and what they provide in terms of products and services. The organizations that survive identify and meet the needs, wants, and priorities of enough people to warrant survival. A customer may be the ultimate user/consumer of a product or service, a purchaser who makes decisions for others, or both a purchaser and a consumer. A customer may be internal to the organization (or "captive"), using the output or services of another department or division, or may be external, choosing among competing organizations to meet their needs, wants, and priorities. The external customer is the subject of this chapter.

Because women make the majority of healthcare decisions and purchases for their families, they are the retail-marketing target for PCPs in support of the entire demand chain. Our first priority, then, is to capture Mrs. Smith and meet all her healthcare needs, wants, and priorities within our demand chain.

Chapter 2 discussed the factors that influence Mrs. Smith's choice of primary care physicians, including geographic access. My consulting firm's zip code analysis of numerous primary care practices verifies that women prefer to develop a relationship with a PCP located reasonably close to their homes. We find that a majority of established primary care patients in urban and suburban areas live within a five-mile to seven-mile radius of their providers. This radius translates to roughly a ten-minute drive in most nonrural communities.

If we want to capture Mrs. Smith and her family, we must ensure that our demand chain has enough affiliated primary care practices in the right locations to provide access to our targeted neighborhoods. This orientation leads to more clinic sites with fewer providers. You may ask, "But isn't this perspective at odds with the notion of larger clinics pursuing economies of scale?" The answer is yes, but we win the primary care game on the revenue side of the income statement. We win by capturing market share. Even solo practices can break even if the provider has captured an adequate share of the market.

Some potential economies exist in sharing a physical plant and equipment across several doctors. Billing software can certainly manage several practices at once. Even a few economies in support staff costs are available for multiple providers in the same location. My team and I insist that our client practices manage their costs according to benchmark ratios, but it is clear to all of us that we cannot "cost cut" our way to success in a poorly performing primary care practice (or specialty practice, for that matter). The largest expense in the small PCP group cost structure is the physician (usually about 50 percent). Yet the physician is also the revenue-generating engine for the practice. Consequently, the greatest potential for performance improvement in the practice is in optimizing the efficiency of the physician. The fundamental requirement for optimization is patient volume— in other words, capturing and servicing market share. Some of the most productive medical practices require more support staff and space per provider rather than less; yet their financial performance is superior to other practices.

Physicians and management should carefully and consistently control costs in a medical practice, but they should not hesitate to sacrifice some on the cost side to be in the right place to capture Mrs. Smith and her neighbors before competitors do so. Of course, this revenue-based strategy assumes that we have done our homework and have placed the practices in locations where there are or will be enough households to support the providers. Otherwise, no amount of advertising or cost cutting will bring the practice to financial viability. (Tactics for addressing geographic locations that are growing but do not yet have the potential patient volume to support a practice are discussed later in this chapter.)

Of course, capturing Mrs. Smith (creating a customer) is only half the objective. We must also keep that customer. A competent physician and her support staff have the competitive advantage when they are the first in a new market. Mrs. Smith prefers not to change providers if she can avoid it. If we can capture her before competing demand chains do, we have established a significant entry barrier for our competitors. Nevertheless, wise providers and demand chains do not leave patient retention to chance. The second half of this chapter addresses the retention component of our fundamental mission.

CONCEPT 2: THE PROCESS OF RETAIL ANALYSIS

As my hospital clients have learned, the process of retail analysis and strategy development is not conceptually complex, but it does take a different mind-set for most hospitals and medical practices, which traditionally have had the "build it and they will come" mentality. Retail analysis requires not only understanding the population within our targeted market(s) but also analyzing our competitors' retail penetration as well as supply and demand data for each primary care specialty. Once this information is collected, capacity needs by specialty will surface, as will strategic needs (locations where plenty of PCPs exist, but they are wearing our competitors' jerseys.) The objectives of retail analysis in the targeted area (usually identified by zip codes) include the following:

- Determine if additional PCPs are needed.
- Determine what type and how many additional PCPs are needed.

- Determine where additional PCPs are needed.
- Determine when additional PCPs will be needed.
- Develop tactics to address the identified retail opportunities.

The analysis process also involves the following steps.

Market Definition

Most hospitals have identified their primary and secondary service areas, often based on the origin of past patients, but medical practices are less likely to do so. The first step in retail analysis is to define the anticipated target market. The definition may be modified as additional demographic analysis is conducted, but having a starting point is essential. Because most of the data analyzed are categorized by zip code and because most urban and suburban areas have multiple zip codes, those zip codes can be used to identify the targeted market.

Demographic Analysis

Once the market has been identified, demographic data can be gathered for the designated zip codes. Sources of demographic data include ESRI (www.esri.com), Claritas (www.claritas.com), and the U.S. Census Bureau (www.census.gov). Analysts should gather a variety of data points to identify current and future population estimates in total and for various age categories (such as under age 18 or over age 55). The analysis should also include indicators of population trends, such as median age of homes in the zip code, average household size, and median household income. I also recommend identifying any significant ethnic groups within the targeted area because properly addressing language and culture issues can enhance a growing practice. A visit to the local chamber of commerce or community department of economic development can yield significant data and insights regarding current and future community growth. All of these factors (and many others) help define community needs and potential opportunities.

Competitor Analysis

An essential component of retail analysis is the identification and documentation of the current geographic retail and other demand-chain locations of competitors. Competitors include hospitals, ambulatory services settings, and employed or affiliated PCPs associated with competing demand chains. Also make note of primary care splitters—those who refer or admit to competing hospitals—along with estimates of the business they do with us versus competing facilities.

Demand-Chain Analysis

Now identify and document the geographic locations of your own affiliated hospitals, affiliated ambulatory services settings, and affiliated and employed PCPs. This step is often more complicated than it may seem, depending on the accuracy of medical staff records.

Provider Capacity Analysis

Document by zip code and drive time the number of primary care physicians in each location and compare these with the current and anticipated population to identify areas of need and surplus by primary care specialty. Organizations such as Solucient and MedStat produce databases that compare age, sex, and other demographic data with the supply of physicians by specialty. These databases are

extremely helpful in identifying physician need or surplus by specialty for defined geographic areas. My firm usually completes this
analysis for the entire market area and population (to assess
whether there is a capacity opportunity or a physician distribution
problem). We also complete the analysis for each zip code to help
assess where needs in one zip code might currently be met by physicians in an adjacent zip code.

Payer Analysis

The next step is to identify major payers operating within the
marketplace, along with any significant negotiating leverage, significant contracts, or other influences that might affect the retail
strategy.

Retail-Corridor Analysis

Certain nonhealthcare retailers have developed sophisticated methods for identifying new locations based on market trends. Those
who have a reasonable record of success in selecting new sites include
Walgreen's, Wal-Mart, CVS, Home Depot, and Target. While these
retailers may be hesitant to share their methods, the results of their
planning ultimately become visible and can validate primary care
site selection based on current and anticipated population trends.

Data Mapping

Once these analyses are complete, document the results by using
mapping software. Several maps help facilitate subsequent tactical
planning sessions. For example, one can use an overlay to show primary care practice locations on current and projected population
densities.

Capacity Opportunities

Once data have been gathered and the mapping is complete, hospital executives and planners can look for obvious opportunities to add physician capacity to the market. Sometimes these capacity opportunities are a function of current demand. However, planners should not overlook the opportunity to "grow" additional primary care capacity as a target population expands, moves, or ages. Capacity opportunities usually rank high on the priority list because they are relatively low risk. Providers who enter a targeted geography that has excess demand may also realize a "first in" advantage, which ultimately may become a significant barrier to entry for other competitors.

Strategic Needs

Retail analysis often identifies certain geographic areas where PCP capacity is adequate or excessive but the physicians all refer to or admit to other demand chains. In this case, hospitals or medical practice executives may still choose to enter the area for strategic reasons. Because of the inherently higher risk of not being the first in the market, the tactics in this scenario will, of necessity, differ from those in market areas where there is excess demand for services.

Strategic Priorities

With data analysis and mapping completed and capacity and strategic targets identified, it is time to prioritize the opportunities. While we can apply mathematical models to the variables, this process is still largely subjective and involves comparing opportunities against factors such as the type of opportunity (capacity or strategic), the presence of other key retailers, the availability of tactical options (e.g., a nearby established practice), anticipated population growth, and anticipated competitor response.

Implementation Tactics

After the targets are identified and prioritized, the final step is to identify the most effective tactics for addressing each retail target. For example, in a target area with excess demand for primary care services, the hospital and its demand-chain partners might choose to open a new practice with three new physicians starting one year apart over three years. In a target area with excess capacity, the hospital might try to acquire an established group practice, employ an established provider or group, or change referral patterns by building relationships between affiliated specialists and the target PCPs. In such instances, analysts should develop a pro forma financial statement for each tactic. The projected costs of each tactic and its potential for success may result in modifications to the strategic priorities already discussed.

The process of retail analysis provides tremendous insight that will inform the strategic and medical staff planning activities undertaken by most hospitals and many larger medical groups. The process also identifies potential tactics for addressing targeted markets.

CONCEPT 3: RETAIL IMPLEMENTATION TACTICS

Tactics for acquiring market share may seem antithetical to the economizing tactics used by many hospitals and medical groups. However, commitment only to controlling expenses frequently results in missed opportunities. Let me explain.

I have seen several hospitals and health systems wake up to find that while they were increasing the efficiency of their primary care practices through site closures and consolidations, their competitors were capturing market share right in their own backyards. My consulting team has been hired to help clients respond to these aggressive competitors—a tough (and expensive) task. On the other hand, other hospitals and health systems have continued to grow their primary care market presence despite the financial commitment involved, and they now dominate in terms of hospital market share. Their competitors are hopelessly playing catch up (and I do mean hopelessly). As long as these dominant players continue to manage their retail relationships, they will continue to own their markets.

Conducting a retail analysis of a targeted geographic market usually yields two types of opportunities:

1. Capacity opportunities are found in geographic areas where the current or anticipated population exceeds or will exceed the current supply of physicians and where excess demand for services is not being met by providers at a location in an adjacent zip code that is within a ten-minute drive of the urban and suburban consumer.
2. Strategic opportunities are found in areas where physician supply is adequate (or even excessive) but the existing physicians are affiliated with another demand chain.

Where excess demand for services exists, the bigger risk is not acting to shore up market share before a competitor does so. On the other hand, when demand is being met, the task of entering a market and creating a viable practice is much more challenging, even if the population is growing. Established providers in the area have the advantage because their current patients serve as a strong sales force, and patients tend to maintain established relationships with their physicians. Most hospitals find themselves facing both capacity and strategic opportunities in markets where competitors are present.

Growing Primary Care Practices

Before developing tactics to address these two types of opportunities, strategists must understand the dynamics of developing a primary care practice. "Mary, Mary, quite contrary, how does your garden grow?" is the question of the day. How does a primary care practice grow, and how can we facilitate that growth to maximize opportunities for success?

The growth rate and viability of a primary care practice are determined by the development of a base of satisfied patients who refer their friends and relatives as opportunities to do so arise. The passive nature of this "sales" or referral process usually results in an extended start-up period (about two years). Appendix B is a pro forma illustrating how a cold-start practice (a practice starting new, with no momentum) might grow during that two-year time frame.

A number of factors affect how quickly a primary care practice will grow, including the following:

- *Physician gender.* Female physicians tend to build practices more quickly than their male counterparts.
- *Physician personality.* An outgoing physician who communicates easily with patients will build a practice more quickly than a physician with a more reserved personality.
- *Physician appearance and demeanor.* A physician who dresses professionally and has a pleasant demeanor will grow a practice more quickly than one who appears sloppy, aloof, or surly.
- *Market demand.* The larger the number of unattached patients and the farther patients must travel to obtain primary medical care, the greater the chance that they will try the new provider and location.
- *Customer service.* New patients often have formed an opinion about a physician well before they actually meet him. Their experiences with the appointment desk staff, the receptionist, and the clinical assistant have already enhanced or tainted their opinion. Before the physician ever enters the examination room, she has been placed on a pedestal or in a pit from which recovery will be difficult at best.
- *Warm start.* A warm start involves adding a new physician to an established practice and taking advantage of the existing patient volume and referral momentum. Such momentum can

dramatically reduce the amount of time it takes to build a viable new practice.

- *Promotional activities.* An effective promotional plan involves appropriate advertising to alert patients to the new practice. Newspaper announcements and mailers are common for most new practices, but they should be only the beginning of promotional activities that will increase the visibility of the physicians in the target marketplace. (Although there are exceptions, patients tend to select primary care physicians rather than practices.) Public-speaking opportunities, teaching opportunities, service opportunities, direct mail, health fairs, sports events, involvement in the Rotary Club, church attendance, and many other factors increase a physician's visibility and marketability.
- *Location.* Medical practices are a destination retail location rather than a convenience retail location (such as a 7-11, Maverick, or Shell convenience store). For this reason, a primary care practice does not need to be "conveniently" located on a corner lot, but reasonable access and visibility from main thoroughfares offer an advantage over being hidden away in a neighborhood.

Armed with a retail strategy and a basic understanding of how primary care practices develop, hospital and physician leaders can identify implementation tactics to achieve their strategic objectives. Although the specifics of implementation may vary significantly by local circumstance, demand chain strategists should take note of several general rules of thumb.

Capacity Opportunities

If a capacity opportunity has been identified, the following tactical questions should be asked:

- Do we have an affiliated and established family practice group nearby that might be expanded to meet the need?

- If we do not have an affiliated group within a reasonable drive time, do any of our established and affiliated physicians draw a number of their patients from the target market area?
- If no proximate established and affiliated group exists, can we recruit the right graduating resident to staff and build a new practice?
- Would on-call coverage be available in the market to support a new physician(s) while we grow the new practice?
- Can we hire support staff for the practice location?
- Is adequate office space (in terms of square footage, cost, location, and so forth) available in the target market area?
- What actions, if any, are our competitors likely to take when they see our entry into the targeted market area?

Strategic Opportunities

Tackling a strategic opportunity is, of course, more challenging than addressing unmet demand in a market area. Adding capacity to a market without excess demand (especially when there is limited hope for population growth) results in a zero-sum game—a potentially expensive proposition for the new practice and the established practices that will share a smaller slice of the same pie. Hospitals are almost always required to employ new strategic PCPs because independent physician groups in the demand chain do not have the capital to endure the financial drain of a lengthy practice start-up. Instead of adding a new physician to meet a strategic opportunity, some demand chains try to attract or even acquire existing capacity in the target market area. This approach can be difficult to implement with established practices and their loyalties, but it can be accomplished with the help of specialty physicians who recognize PCPs as customers. I have had the experience of attracting specialty referrals across town, against migration patterns, to the smaller hospital with the help of surgeons who spent a little bit of time over dinner building new PCP relationships—an illustration of the power of an effective demand chain.

Family Medicine

Because of family practitioners' ability to provide service to the entire age spectrum, the family medicine specialty is well suited to capture market share in urban, suburban, and rural settings. Other primary care specialties are essential to the demand chain but are not as well suited for capturing families in these settings. Many general internists prefer to locate closer to a hospital campus where they can build an inpatient component of their practice. Obstetricians tend to locate within a short distance of the hospital because they need reasonable access to labor and delivery as well as surgical suites. If pediatric inpatient services are part of the demand chain, pediatricians are a great addition to a retail strategy in urban and suburban settings. (If a children's hospital is nearby, most demand chains cede pediatrics to these specialized delivery networks.) Once family practices are established, adding other primary care specialties (and rotating other subspecialists through the established practices) helps to target patients based on specific needs identified in the captured market.

Capacity Timing

Regardless of the primary care specialty or the opportunity, the ideal approach is to recruit one new physician to the target market (cold or warm start) and allow that practice to gain momentum for several months before adding more physician capacity. Adding multiple new physicians to a single practice location simultaneously is a prescription for extended financial losses and physician frustration, unless there is significant unmet demand for services in the area. Two new physicians added to a location will not double the patient volume flowing to the new practice. Instead, it will usually halve the number of patients that would otherwise be seen by a single new provider. The rest of the time will be spent with these expensive resources twiddling their thumbs. Again, depending on the circumstances, I often recommend at least a year interval between each addition of new capacity to a practice.

Bricks and Mortar

Many hospitals have been quick to build new facilities to accommodate new practices (sometimes at twice the cost per square foot paid by private practices), thinking that having a new facility will somehow stake their claim to the market. My colleagues and I usually counsel our clients to spend their capital adding primary care capacity rather than bricks and mortar to the market. Capture the market share by leasing accessible storefronts or other freestanding facilities and adding providers over time. Once the market share is captured and the needs, wants, and priorities of the patient/customer base are identified, plan a new facility with the right specialty mix and the right diagnostic capabilities in the right location. This approach will ensure that the beautiful new building will not sit empty waiting for new practices to grow, while financial losses mount and board members and senior managers lose confidence and withdraw their support.

The development and implementation of a primary care retail strategy is usually driven and funded by the hospital. In addition to capturing and retaining market share in primary care practices, hospital and demand chain strategists must also pay close attention to keeping that market share within the demand chain by attracting appropriate referrals from PCPs. This will be the subject of Chapter 8.

Living or Dying by Referrals

This chapter presents four concepts:

- Referrals drive the healthcare business
- The referral management challenge
- Relationship management
- Demand-chain management

CONCEPT 1: REFERRALS DRIVE THE HEALTHCARE BUSINESS

I was visiting with several acquaintances in the restaurant business. They had just returned from an annual corporate conference in Las Vegas. During the course of our conversation, they mentioned the lavish dinner they had on the last evening of their trip, paid for by one of their suppliers. Shortly thereafter, I was bombarded with one of those painful but ever-present auto-dealer radio advertisements emphasizing dealer incentives. Next I stopped at the home of my good friend, a consumer electronics salesman, who has a beautiful house (paid for by commissions) that is furnished with several "gifts" he won from manufacturers or suppliers for selling a particular name brand. Even my own small consulting firm wisely hired a superb sales executive who receives a base salary and a commission directly tied to the amount of new business she brings to our organization.

In most business enterprises, creating and keeping customers involves incentives, discounts, favors, meals, commissions, gifts, trips, and other perks. Those who seek out or refer business are rewarded, often handsomely, for their work because they have generated an immediate downstream effect on an entire supply chain. In addition, exclusivity agreements often keep that captured business within a specific supply chain and become fodder for lawsuits if they are violated.

The business of healthcare (which must also create and keep a customer) is different. Incentives, discounts, favors, meals, commissions, gifts, and trips will result in huge financial penalties and potentially a lot of time in a small space to reflect on life. Terms such as "anti-kickback," "inurement," "private benefit," and "the Stark Law" are a source of significant confusion and significant legal fees. Everyone has an anecdote about a brush with the Internal Revenue Service, the Office of the Inspector General, or an aggressive state attorney general, and of course the stories get better with every telling. Becoming the subject of an investigation is a huge issue, and organizations and individuals are assumed to be guilty unless and until they are proven innocent. This threat alone is a great deterrent for most of my clients. It is not uncommon for the mere mention of the term "referral" to cause meeting participants to glance at each other nervously, close doors, and check each other's identification tags.

My intent here is not to question the purpose or value of government regulation in healthcare. Medicare and Medicaid dollars (my taxes) should be protected from abusive business practices. And patients should be protected from abusive referrals for unnecessary services or to inferior providers of services for a fee or kickback. Greed and avarice have no place in organizations and relationships that influence patients' lives.

Nevertheless, and despite the regulations, referrals drive the health-care business. The majority of new patients who contact a primary care practice are referred by a friend or relative who is already a patient at the practice. The majority of referrals to specialty physicians come from primary care physicians. The majority of referrals for ancillary services and drugs require a doctor's order or prescription (a referral form). Few hospital executives would want to live only on the inpatient business coming through their emergency departments. Without referrals from primary care and specialty physicians, hospitals would be out of business in short order and hospital-based physicians would be retraining. Referrals are essential in healthcare because patients/customers do not have the ability to navigate the demand chain on their own—even with the Internet! Winning referrals must be a critical focus for every member of every demand chain, because without an adequate number of them there is no demand chain and no practice. Just ask a small community that has closed its hospital or lost its only local physician.

The key, of course, is how we attract referrals to our practice, our diagnostic imaging center, our hospital, and our demand chain.

Previous chapters discussed the retail customer, the role of primary care providers in capturing and retaining customers, the demand chain, and the roles played by PCPs, specialists, hospitals, and hospital-based physicians in moving and keeping market share within the demand chain. Patient/customer referrals are the current that flows up (and sometimes down) a properly functioning demand chain, benefiting all demand chain members in the process. Managing that current and avoiding a break in the circuitry (the loss of a referral to a competitor) is the subject of this chapter.

CONCEPT 2: THE REFERRAL MANAGEMENT CHALLENGE

With the exception of PCPs and a few internal medicine subspecialties, most members of the medical services demand chain do not capture and retain market share. Hospitals, hospital-based specialists, diagnostic imaging centers, specialty physicians, and any other non-PCPs must attract referrals to survive. Most do so legally by trying to provide a great workshop, consistent clinical quality, and superior service to patients and referring physicians.

Still, in most markets, many of these critical referral relationships are left to chance rather than being managed proactively. Sure, the hospital CEO meets with medical staff leaders and top-producing surgeons. Senior executives meet with the physicians who support their assigned hospital service lines, but few hospitals or physicians have a comprehensive process in place to develop and cement relationships up and down the demand chain. Importantly, few demand chains have any forum to actively unify and focus their combined efforts on better meeting the needs, wants, and priorities of the retail and demand-chain customers who are so critical to their success.

Consider the potential for a group of demand-chain leaders with a vision to move their market share from 40 percent to 50 percent over a three-year period. The group consists of physician leaders from the departments of radiology, pathology, anesthesiology, and emergency. The hospitalists and intensivists are also represented. The group also includes physician leaders from the demand chain's key service lines, including general surgery, orthopedics, cardiology, obstetrics, and oncology. The hospital CEO is a charter member, as are a few key executives. Lastly, the group includes physician leaders from internal medicine, family medicine, and potentially pediatrics. (This sounds a bit like a medical staff, doesn't it?)

The group's charter is clear. It is focused on better understanding the needs, wants, and priorities of the retail customer—Mrs. Smith. The group meets frequently to hear from internal and outside experts about the latest market research on Mrs. Smith and her needs. (The challenge of engaging busy physicians in "one more meeting" is examined later in this chapter.) The group also discusses the latest results of the focus groups they jointly sponsor to better understand both patients and buyers of medical care. The group has a common patient satisfaction measurement process and openly shares and discusses the results from the hospital, hospital-based specialty physicians, and individual ambulatory medical practices. Members with the strongest scores discuss their best practices with those who have not yet reached perfection. They talk to one another to better understand the needs, wants, and priorities of each demand-chain member. They jointly develop tactics, commit to action plans, and share best practices, both giving and receiving critical customer feedback. As a result, the demand chain outperforms every other organization in its marketplace, even the fully integrated model.

Is this demand-chain scenario impossible? No! Is it improbable if not formally managed? Absolutely! Is this level of alignment easy or quick to achieve? Not a chance! That is why those who achieve anything close to this level of demand-chain management have a sustainable strategic advantage over their competitors.

Is this model illegal? Is it illegal to have the most responsive radiologists in town, always anxious to meet the needs of referring physicians and their patients? Is it illegal to provide the best-equipped and most efficient surgical suites, the finest anesthesiologists, and the most skilled nursing staff in the area to facilitate the surgeons' productivity and ability to practice their profession? Is it illegal for specialists to treat primary care physicians as customers to attract their business? Is there anything illegal about high-quality clinical care and superb customer service?

Is this a Pollyanna scenario? I do not believe so. In fact, I believe it is the way the business of medicine should be conducted. Can I point to anyone who has fully achieved this vision in today's tough environment? No. Can I point to anyone who has proven that the theory works? You bet, and so can you. Think of the general surgeon who personally calls the referring physician to discuss the disposition of each case and confer about follow-up. Think of the service-line executive and physician leaders who meet with every PCP in town to solicit their input regarding the product line. Think of the obstetrician who travels to a rural community each month to assist family practitioners with high-risk obstetrics patients and gynecology issues. Think of the radiologists who fast-track every referring physician request. Are these not all examples of the very concepts we have been discussing?

Granted, the barriers to this level of demand-chain integration are myriad, making it that much more difficult to achieve, but it is also that much more sustainable. The following barriers come to mind:

- Some of our potential demand-chain members are opening their own surgery centers or diagnostic centers.
- Some of our medical staff members do not even speak to each other, let alone work together with the hospital to achieve some greater purpose.
- Our affiliated doctors are too busy with their own issues to worry about the bigger picture.
- Some of our specialists are splitters who work, out of necessity or otherwise, with our competing hospital.
- Some of our physicians are members of a large multispecialty group that works to keep its referrals within its own group rather than support the general medical staff.

Few demand chains are even close to perfect. Nevertheless, every hospital and some of its affiliated physicians can begin to improve their focus on their retail customers and each other. Start small, but start somewhere!

CONCEPT 3: RELATIONSHIP MANAGEMENT

Building relationships among physicians and between physicians and the hospital is the key to managing the demand chain. Actively maintaining those relationships is even more critical and more difficult in an environment in which members of the hospital's medical staff can so easily become the hospital's competitors.

In the late 1980s and early 1990s many hospitals established a position called "physician liaison." The liaison role was intended to build relationships with physicians and their office staffs in an attempt to attract their business to the hospital. Many patterned their approach after drug company representatives, dropping in on offices and giving away pens, notepads, and T-shirts bearing the hospital logo. Some liaisons gathered intelligence from the offices they visited regarding the performance of hospital departments and then passed that information on to hospital executives. A few attempted to "consult" with their assigned medical offices to help them improve their operations. However, most of these early physician liaisons failed to generate much return on their efforts, and this "program of the month" died within a few years.

The physician liaison concept was not wrong. Drug companies have proven its viability over many years. Rather, the implementation of the concept was not effective for the following reasons:

- *Most hospitals did not recognize the liaison role as a sales position and failed to hire sales professionals as liaisons.* Sales professionals know how to gain access to physicians, to build relationships with physicians and their office staffs, to listen for opportunities and challenges, and to drive their organizations to respond to those opportunities. The best sales professionals are organized to a fault, are articulate communicators, and are as tenacious as bulldogs. They know their customers and understand their needs, wants, and priorities so they can match their "wares" to meet those needs, wants, and priorities. They know how to overcome barriers to success in their target organizations and in their own companies to achieve the desired objective.
- *Sales management is both an art and a science.* Successful sales management requires the identification of realistic performance targets, continuous training, dogged motivation, and constant follow-up and accountability. Most hospital executives were unprepared to provide effective sales management because they did not understand the sales process themselves.
- *Many executive teams were unprepared to effectively manage the limited intelligence they received from their liaisons, particularly*

regarding concerns about hospital departments or services.
They made the fundamental relationship-management error
of asking for physician input and then failing to do
anything with that input. This failure to act or communicate with physicians undermined the physician liaison and
caused greater damage than if they had not asked for input
in the first place.

Relationship management in today's environment requires
much more than pens and T-shirts. It requires the commitment and
personal involvement of the hospital CEO, the senior leadership
team, and physician leaders all along the demand chain. And it may
also require a skilled sales professional to ensure the long-term viability of the relationship-management process.

Relationship Management and the Demand Chain

The first principle of demand-chain management is this: Referrals
follow relationships. This simple principle is already being applied
in every healthcare market. Specialists serving rural areas understand
that if they show up once a week or twice a month at the small critical access hospital 30 miles from their main office and spend an
afternoon seeing patients in a satellite office, they will get referrals
from the family practitioners in town. Wise tertiary hospital executives promote such behavior because they know that while simple
surgeries may be performed at the small hospital, the more complex
cases will find their way back to the specialist's main office and to
her preferred hospital.

The same principle applies in large metropolitan areas. PCPs
tend to refer their patients to specialists with whom they have a relationship, which may have started during a residency training program or resulted from a referral through a physician partner. Both
specialists and primary care physicians refer to the hospital where
they have a preferred relationship, which provides an opportunity

for hospital-based physicians to shine. In fact, this referral process is what creates the demand chain in the first place. Again, referrals follow relationships.

The second principle of demand-chain management is this: All relationships atrophy over time. Relationships that are left unattended or that are taken for granted become vulnerable over time. Small frustrations can creep into otherwise healthy relationships, slowly festering below the surface until they become irreconcilable differences. Partners can become so busy that they fail to engage in the niceties—like a thank-you letter or a phone call—that built their referral relationship in the first place. Small offenses or misunderstandings wedge their way into otherwise healthy associations, creating barriers to open communication. Before long, relationships are compromised and vulnerable to attack from outside influences peddling an alternative—sometimes any alternative.

The first step in building a successful demand chain is to develop and maintain relationships among physicians and between physicians and hospital management. Demand-chain leaders must formally and continuously pursue the relationship-management process.

The most likely demand-chain "integrator" (a word that has fallen on hard times but is still descriptive) is the hospital, with its role as the gathering place for the medical staff and with its ability to amass or borrow large amounts of capital (relative to medical practices). The hospital chief executive, as the board-appointed fiduciary, is the driver of this relationship development/management process and must be personally involved in its implementation (Conner 1992). In fact, from a demand-chain management perspective, the hospital CEO has two key responsibilities. The first is relationship development/management. The second is balancing the various demands for capital through appropriate prioritization. All other operating demands can and should be left to qualified daily operations officers.

A successful relationship development and management process in today's more competitive environment is likely to involve a sales professional, but only as an adjunct to a hospital CEO and senior leadership team who are fully engaged in its implementation. Each member of the executive team has assigned responsibilities as part of the organization's relationship-management team. The relationship development and management process is fairly straightforward and includes the following six steps:

1. *Understand the context.* A fundamental challenge for relationship managers is to understand the context and perspective of their target audience—the physician. Hospital executives often communicate with physicians in terms of what is good for the hospital—its mission, values, and challenges. As lofty as that mission and those values may be, most independent medical practices operate somewhere near the bottom of Maslow's hierarchy of needs (Certo 1997). Of necessity, the major concern of independent physicians is meeting their biweekly payroll, covering their monthly mortgage, and figuring out how to fund a retirement plan. Few physicians are self-actualized; their greatest concerns relate to daily operations issues that affect their ability to practice medicine as they see fit. Employed physicians worry (I hope) about the financial performance issues common to hospital-owned practices and whether they will be employed next year. Building a relationship with these demand-chain partners starts with understanding their world and their worries.

2. *Contact customer.* No relationship can be built without taking the risk of "getting dirty." A few CEOs hide from their medical staff members to avoid complaints, conflicts, or having to say "no." Others delegate physician issues to ill-prepared assistant administrators who run interference and serve as convenient scapegoats. These executives are rarely successful at either hiding or remaining employed over the long term. Other CEOs think that an occasional appearance at a medical staff meeting or other formal function constitutes relationship development and management. But relationships

are not built with groups, they are built with individuals. The successful CEO relationship managers not only have an open-door policy with physicians but also target and seek out physicians with whom they can and do build relationships. Some contacts should be formally planned, such as a meal, a face-to-face meeting, or a golf game. Others should be informal, such as meeting in the hallway or in the physician's lounge. Whether formal or informal, such contacts are always purposeful. Customer contacts should periodically occur on the customer's turf. Visiting the medical office (without the pens or T-shirts) sends a powerful message to the targeted physician(s). Site visits are particularly critical in settings where hospitalist programs have reduced or eliminated the need for primary care physicians to frequent the hospital.

In addition to the CEO, the entire leadership team and key physician leaders should also actively participate in relationship development/management. The relationship management team should formally identify their targeted physicians and use a sales database software package, such as ACT!, to assign target contacts, assign relationship managers, and record results. Some physicians may require a quarterly visit. Others may be seen formally only twice a year. Some will be contacted every month, either formally or informally, but always with a purpose.

3. *Listen for opportunity.* The purpose of every contact (formal or otherwise) is to listen to the physician. Stephen Covey (2004, 153) refers to this process as "listening to understand." A few key questions to the physician about his patients and about the practice or the hospital's level of service will likely start the conversation. Every nugget—particularly, negative statements that are difficult to hear—should be carefully explored and documented (usually after the conversation, to permit active listening). The more specific the physician is willing to be, the better. Relationship managers learn that such open

communication may require several contacts, but eventually it will occur. Positive or negative, the feedback should be carefully documented in a contact or sales report and reviewed by the senior leadership team. These sales reports should be considered confidential; they are not intended for wide distribution but are for members of the team who can address the identified issues.

4. *Educate.* After listening carefully for opportunities and restating the physician's comments to ensure understanding, the relationship manager might also share pertinent information with the doctor. Such information may include new services or process improvements that will be of interest to the physician. The information should always include feedback regarding previous discussions and actions that have been taken to address issues identified by the physician or her peers. Once the relationship has been built, educational information might include personal performance feedback from other demand-chain members. Again, the physician's response to educational information should always be a part of the sales or contact reporting process.

5. *Deliver.* Every issue raised by a physician (a demand-chain member) is an opportunity to improve relationships, particularly if the feedback results in improved processes or service to the physician and his peers. (Even if the answer to the physician's request is no, the relationship can be strengthened, particularly if the answer is well supported and is delivered personally from the CEO to the physician. After all, physicians, like everyone else, generally appreciate being heard.) Delivering requires an active review of each sales report to identify issues and opportunities, which should remain on an action agenda until they are resolved. Progress on action agenda items should be reviewed as a critical part of every senior leadership meeting with the CEO, who should hold her direct reports accountable for delivering results in a timely manner.

6. *Follow up.* Providing formal feedback to the physician regarding the disposition of her issues or requests is an essential part of building and maintaining relationships. Such feedback also provides a legitimate purpose for another contact. Thank-you notes, letters, or other small tokens of appreciation are good ways to acknowledge suggestions that yield improved processes. I also recommend that the CEO be personally involved in follow-up, especially when the answer to the physician's request is negative.

Establishing a formal relationship-management process is a significant undertaking, but it can produce tremendous results. The relationships, communication, and trust that develop are an essential prerequisite to developing a strong demand chain.

CONCEPT 4: DEMAND-CHAIN MANAGEMENT

Demand-chain management is a process, not an event. It is not brought about by fiat or formal announcement. Rather, it is built on a foundation of strong relationships developed and maintained over time. With that foundation in place or developing, management of the demand chain can begin. A good idea is to start small with a select group of demand-chain members who have a common interest and are already predisposed toward clinical and service excellence. For example, a distinct service line is a good potential starting point. The demand-chain management process has six steps:

1. *Ask, "What is working?"* Identify a few specialty and primary care physicians or small medical groups who are already committed to the hospital and to their referral sources and who are willing to provide honest feedback about the hospital and the physicians to whom they refer (including hospital-based physicians). The physicians or groups you identify may be hospital-based, employed, or independent, but they should be

well respected clinically and politically among medical staff members. Talk to these physicians about their needs, wants, and priorities related to the selected service line, and document the results. Consider questions such as the following:

- How did they develop their current physician referral patterns?
- Why do they continue to use the physicians to whom they refer?
- What do they expect in terms of access to the physicians to whom they refer?
- What do they expect in terms of feedback from the physicians to whom they refer?
- What kind of feedback do they receive from patients regarding the physicians to whom they refer?
- What has caused them to stop referring to certain physicians in the past?

Similar questions can be asked about the hospital inpatient, outpatient, and diagnostic services as well as those offered by competitors. Responses should be treated confidentially, but the results should be shared with service-line members.

2. *Engage the service-line physicians.* Engage the selected service-line physicians in a dialog and in education regarding retail strategy and demand-chain management. Solicit their support of the hospital's retail strategy and their commitment to participate actively in demand-chain management within their service line. Physicians who are not comfortable with making a commitment to participate should be encouraged to wait until they are willing to make a full commitment.

3. *Establish a demand-chain meeting.* Initiate a 90-minute meeting one evening each month with the engaged physicians. The purposes of the meeting are to continue demand-chain education; receive feedback from physicians interviewed in step 1; review service performance for all members of the demand

chain (the hospital should review its performance improvement action plans and progress with the group); increase the group's understanding of retail and demand-chain customer needs, wants, and priorities; and share best practices among attendees.

4. *Measure performance.* Work with the engaged physicians to develop service measurement tools for retail customers and for other members of the demand chain. Rigorously measure performance on both fronts, and report that performance openly during the monthly demand-chain meeting.

5. *Improve performance.* Commit to performance improvement throughout the demand chain, regardless of areas of identified weakness. This objective may be accomplished with the support of a hospital-sponsored professional services group consisting of education or consulting resources available at a reasonable cost. Physician offices involved in the service line may also share resources with one another.

6. *Broaden physician membership.* Approach additional physicians to assess their willingness to participate actively in demand-chain management. Success breeds success. As one service line succeeds in improving its service and reputation, select another service line and share the principles of success.

Overcoming the Barriers

Active participation in the demand chain is a privilege available to every willing physician—that is, every physician who is willing to commit to the success of the demand chain and to the effort required to actively participate. Remember, the purpose of the demand chain is to attract market share captured in your affiliated primary care practices to your affiliated specialty physicians and to your affiliated hospital and its service lines. Cooperation among all members of the demand chain will lead to an increase in (and retention of) the size of your share of the pie. Success also increases the capital available in the hospital workshop for state-of-the-art facilities, equipment, clinical services, services for the uninsured and underserved, and medical staff development.

But what about the reality of barriers to physician participation in the demand chain? What about those who have opened ambulatory surgery centers or freestanding diagnostic centers? Let's face it: they are competitors. Yes, they may be important customers of the hospital and our affiliated specialists, and we hope to keep as much of their business as possible (and they should hope to keep as much of our referral business as possible), but they are clearly competing with us. They may be the only physician or group in a particular specialty. If so, they will continue to receive our demand-chain business unless or until we can justify an alternative. But our affiliated PCPs should encourage them to support our affiliated specialists and our affiliated capital-generating engine—the hospital—with referred patients. While this may seem like a hard-line approach, it is really no different than physicians choosing to compete with our demand chain in the first place. It levels the playing field.

What about the common communication challenges among physicians and between physicians and management? Groups consisting of physicians and management should consider participating in "crucial conversations" training to help them improve their ability to deal with situations in which the stakes are high, opinions are strongly held, and personal risk exists (Patterson et al. 2002). This training establishes the rules of the game for effective communication during formal demand-chain meetings as well as during information exchanges among demand-chain members.

What about physicians who are too busy to participate? Again, hospital executives must understand that all a physician has to sell is her time. Every hour spent in a meeting or a conversation has a significant opportunity cost in terms of revenue generation and personal recovery or family time. The independent physician's payroll never takes a payday off. He usually does not have capital reserves to facilitate risk taking. The invitation to participate in the demand chain should be sensitive to these circumstances. Meetings should be held after normal office hours and should start and conclude on time. Minutes of the meetings should be made available to members who miss an occasional meeting, although participation is clearly part of the commitment. If some physicians are just not able to make the commitment at the present time, be patient. Let the positive impressions of engaged peers influence the nonparticipants over time.

What about specialists who split their work between two hospitals? This is a tougher situation to manage, particularly if the specialty has limited availability and call coverage reinforces such splitting. Keeping the service "in town" is usually the first priority. The second priority is to attract as much of the business as possible to our demand chain. Becoming the specialty physician partner of choice may involve purposeful workshop or service-line strategies to make our demand chain more valuable to the splitter. It will also usually involve controlling enough of the market share in affiliated primary care practices so that the specialist's interests are aligned with those of our demand-chain members. Splitters who favor our demand chain can be very effective demand-chain members.

Then there is the large multispecialty group across the street from the hospital. They account for a large percentage of our inpatient and outpatient business, but they also compete with us in terms of laboratory, radiology, and other diagnostic services. They make some of the smaller independent specialists nervous because of their affiliated PCPs. Large multispecialty groups are a huge potential advantage if they are aligned with the interests of the hospital and other members of the medical staff. When they are not aligned, they represent a significant potential liability and competition. Large groups already have the potential advantage of aligned incentives, and if they have a number of primary care physician members, they may own or control a large market share. They may aggressively direct patient referrals to their affiliated specialists and to their own ancillary services. This is where relationship development/management becomes so critical. Working to align and maintain relationships with a well-managed multispecialty group is much easier than aligning a number of independent physicians and small groups to compete with the larger group practice.

Every market is different, yet every market can support some level of demand-chain development and management. The more integrated the demand-chain members become in their focus on capturing and retaining market share, the more sustainable will be their competitive advantage. Hospitals that have successfully entered the primary care business and that employ several primary care physicians to support their service lines and affiliated specialty physicians have a distinct advantage in demand-chain development and management. They also have a distinct advantage in overcoming the barriers to demand-chain integration.

Again, developing and managing an effective demand chain for even a single service line is certainly a challenge. It takes great leadership (both clinical and administrative), great relationships and trust, and a commitment to growing the whole pie as well as individual pieces of that pie. It takes tremendous effort and commitment to a formal process. It takes a bit of humility, a lot of tolerance for different viewpoints, and even a bit of luck. Once achieved, however, demand-chain momentum is difficult for even the most astute competitor to circumvent—hence, the sustainability of the demand chain.

REFERENCES

Certo, S. C. 1997. *Supervision: Quality, Diversity, and Technology, 2nd ed.* New York: McGraw-Hill.

Conner, D. R. 1992. *Managing at the Speed of Change.* New York: Villard Books.

Covey, S. R. 2004. *The 8th Habit: From Effectiveness to Greatness.* New York: The Free Press.

Patterson, K., J. Grenny, R. McMillan, A. Switzler, and S. Covey. 2002. *Crucial Conversations: Tools for Talking When Stakes Are High.* New York: McGraw-Hill.

CHAPTER 9

Other Significant Influences on the Demand Chain

This chapter presents two concepts:

- Primary influences
- Secondary influences

The way market share is captured and retained within the demand chain is illustrated in its simplest terms in the demand-chain model in Figure 5. In reality, the healthcare industry is not so simple. The demand chain does not operate in a vacuum, and many factors affect its implementation in any given location or community. Primary influences directly affect the way the demand chain works, while secondary influences indirectly affect the demand chain and the industry. Ignorance of or refusal to acknowledge these influences places the demand chain and its members at significant risk.

CONCEPT 1: PRIMARY INFLUENCES

Primary influences on the demand chain—those that directly affect its operation—include third-party payers and reimbursement, regulators

Figure 5. Medical Services Demand Chain

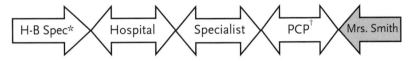

* Hospital-based specialist
† Primary care provider

and their enforcement arms, complementary and alternative medicine practitioners, and the community/population itself.

Third-Party Payers

A fascinating characteristic of the healthcare industry is that Mrs. Smith, who selects healthcare services for her family, might not actually pay for the goods and services she chooses—at least not directly—or she might pay only a small portion of the bill. Mrs. Smith is likely to be insured through a commercial insurer or through participation in a government program such as Medicare or Medicaid. Like other insurers, these programs are based on actuarially determined probabilities. They gather money in the form of insurance premiums or allocated tax revenue to cover the estimated risk of healthcare costs for a defined population. If the costs have been properly estimated, if utilization of services is appropriate, and if the commercial payer has done an adequate job of negotiating fees with physicians and hospitals, the payer will have enough revenue to (1) pay the providers according to the fee schedule (sometimes called the "medical loss ratio," which is an interesting concept in and of itself), (2) cover its own sales and administrative costs, and (3) turn a profit for its investors. If government programs have been equally successful at estimating demand for medical services, adequate revenue will be available. If not, the programs will operate at a deficit, further burdening state and federal budgets. The underlying motivation for commercial payers and government legislators is to reduce costs and limit utilization. A few of the tactics commonly used to lower the medical loss ratio are reducing provider reimbursement, capitation (or "decapitation," as it is sometimes called), preauthorization, and authorized drug formularies.

"When the pie shrinks, the table manners change." I do not know the source of this quotation, but it is certainly apropos to this discussion. The shrinking pie that results from decreasing reimbursement challenges the relationships that are essential to the success of demand chains. Those who pay for healthcare services have the incentive and larger buyers have the power or ability to control (that is, reduce) the amount they pay for the services provided by demand-chain members. As actual income and potential income shrink for all members of the demand chain, individual efforts to sustain personal compensation, cover overhead, and accumulate capital have come under tremendous pressure. Most demand-chain members are working harder to stay even, or are making or accumulating less than just a few years ago. Scarcity has replaced the abundance mentality of earlier days (Covey 1989). Some would say that greed has driven the response of demand-chain members, who are now more likely to do battle than to cooperate. Certainly, greed may play a role with some, but I believe the vast majority of demand-chain members are reacting to this perceived scarcity out of fear rather than greed. Fear, of course, is a survival emotion, which in its lowest form focuses human energy on self-preservation—quite contrary to a healthy demand chain.

Although millions of U.S. citizens do not have medical insurance coverage, the majority of the population in any community does participate in a commercial or government medical insurance program of some type (DeNavas-Walt, Proctor, and Lee 2005). Demand-chain members who desire to provide medical services must therefore negotiate with at least the larger payers to have access to most of the population. Very few providers in very

Figure 6. Payers as "Filter" Along the Medical Services Demand Chain

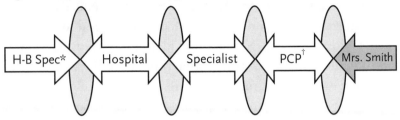

* Hospital-based specialist
† Primary care provider
Ovals represent payers

few communities can survive financially if they ignore any significant payer. Consequently, payers serve as a type of filter for patient access to each provider along the demand chain (Figure 6). Demand-chain participants, particularly PCPs, may be able to leverage the strength of the demand chain in negotiating fees and other terms with payers. However, the primary purpose of the demand chain is to capture and retain market share in primary care practices and to attract that market share to affiliated specialists and to the hospital, which is the capital-generating engine within the demand chain. Thus, the demand chain must negotiate with payers for reasonable reimbursement and access to potential patients for all members.

Regulators and Their Enforcement Arms

In addition to paying the largest portion of the healthcare bill, Uncle Sam is also a legislator, a regulator, a police officer, and a taxing agent. In each of these roles, the government has a direct influence on the operations of the demand chain. Through the use of laws and regulations, legislators attempt to protect the public and to prevent fraudulent and unethical business practices within the healthcare community. In fulfilling their oversight responsibility for the nation's largest payer, legislators also approve plans proposed by the Centers for Medicare and Medicaid Services to control the nation's healthcare bill by reducing reimbursement for providers serving Medicare or Medicaid patients. Both state and federal policing agents ensure compliance with laws and regulations and investigate organizations and individuals suspected of violating policy. Potential consequences for such violations include exclusion from government payer programs, fines for individuals and organizations, loss of tax-exempt status (for those so blessed), and jail time. Our nation's legislators and regulators also, over time, close loopholes in current laws and regulations. In addition, our courts continue to clarify the rule of law as providers are brought to task by the Office of Inspector General, the Internal Revenue Service, state attorneys general, and other enforcement arms.

The current and potential impact of these various legal/regulatory influences on the demand chain is beyond the scope of this text. However, even laypersons can recognize the importance of avoiding any hint of a direct or indirect kickback to members of the demand chain for their referrals. In addition, particularly as the demand chain matures and becomes increasingly integrated, members should be alert to activities that would hamper competition in the marketplace and violate antitrust laws. As always, engaging qualified and thoughtful legal counsel is critical in any strategic activity. (By "thoughtful" I specifically mean someone who is willing to think through the issues at hand rather than hiding behind "no" as a response to any new concept.)

Complementary and Alternative Medicine Practitioners

During most of our discussion of "retail" physician specialties, we have focused on the four primary care specialties: family medicine, general internal medicine, pediatrics, and obstetrics/gynecology. (In many markets these days, both medical doctors and osteopathic physicians in these primary care specialties share after-hours call and work side by side in group practices.) In most markets, however, other retail players can provide healthcare services to many Mrs. Smiths and their families. Some of these providers are complementary to physicians and hospitals. Optometrists, for example, are clearly primary healthcare providers who capture and retain market share. Podiatrists routinely provide both medical and surgical services and are on the medical staffs of many hospitals. Nurse practitioners and physician assistants are offered as complementary alternatives to physicians in many primary care practices and leverage the time of specialty physicians by providing primary medical services in many types of specialty practices. In more rural settings, nurse practitioners and physician assistants may be the only PCPs in the community.

In addition to the complementary providers who are accepted by the general medical community, many other healthcare providers are accepted as legitimate by the ultimate judge—that is, Mrs. Smith—although they might be viewed skeptically by the medical community. Chiropractors, for example, provide spinal manipulation and encourage nutrition as a proven solution for many patient ailments. Chiropractors are found in most communities of any appreciable size. They capture and retain market share because they offer symptom relief for a variety of ailments. Other alternative providers include acupuncturists, naturalists, and massage therapists, all of whom capture a certain market share and potentially serve as referral sources for a demand chain that is wise enough to connect with and educate them. Some mainstream medical providers will say that connecting with an alternative provider might appear to legitimize their services. Thoughtful providers will realize that the Mrs. Smiths captured by alternative providers already consider those providers to be legitimate based on their own experience. The demand chain has nothing to lose and everything to gain by connecting with the alternative provider and being readily available to meet Mrs. Smith's additional needs, wants, and priorities. Both

Figure 7. Medical Services Demand Chain, with Alternative and Complementary Providers

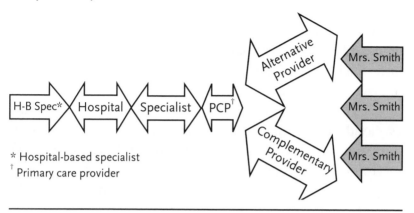

* Hospital-based specialist
† Primary care provider

complementary and alternative providers influence the demand chain (Figure 7).

Community Demographics

Another direct influence on our simple demand-chain model is the large number of Mrs. Smiths and their households that form the community we define as our target market. Community characteristics have a tremendous influence on the demand chain, starting with the word-of-mouth referrals that build most primary care practices. Word of mouth also influences local residents' opinions about the hospital(s) in town. When it comes to hospitals, every community is a hotbed of perspective and opinion, often based on limited anecdotes that become increasingly inaccurate as time goes on. Physicians and medical groups can experience similar image-maintaining challenges, particularly in smaller communities with fewer options.

Other demographic characteristics can have a dramatic influence on the success or failure of a demand chain. For example, hospitals and specialists who fail to position their affiliated PCPs in the faster-growing parts of town may find that they are increasingly isolated as new suburbs attract the younger, well-employed, and well-insured families that are required to support a viable payer mix. Isolated inner-city hospitals face a tremendous struggle to remain financially viable on a diet of Medicaid reimbursement and payments from uninsured patients. Maintaining a viable medical staff becomes increasingly problematic over time as new physicians are attracted to newer facilities and safer patient populations in newer parts of town. Population growth trends; the number of Medicare, Medicaid, and uninsured patients; the general health status of the community; and the age and sex of the population all influence the success of individual providers and entire demand chains. Consequently, the primary care retail strategy associated with the demand chain is critical to the ultimate success or failure of the chain and its individual members.

CONCEPT 2: SECONDARY INFLUENCES

Secondary influences affect not only healthcare but all industries, including the demand chain and its members. Chief among these influences are technology and technological advances; national, state, and local political trends; sociocultural trends; and the economy.

Technology and Technological Advances

Who can deny the impact of technology on every aspect of our business and our lives? Naturally, technology both facilitates and frustrates our efforts to create and maintain a demand chain. On the positive side, the ability to electronically store and communicate everything from basic messages to lab results and diagnostic images provides a tremendous opportunity for demand-chain members to communicate with their respective customers. Demand-chain members can facilitate patient education, send reminders, and offer general practice information to patients who are interested in an electronic communication medium. Among themselves, demand-chain members can share test results, efficiently tap massive clinical databases, and communicate regarding patient diagnoses and treatment protocols. Technology can improve their ability to code and document their services as well as to improve safety in prescribing medications. A shared electronic medical record opens up numerous opportunities to provide highly coordinated care. A few practices are experimenting with patients scheduling their own appointments electronically. The possibilities seem to be endless.

Other positive effects of technology include the availability of increasingly effective diagnostic and therapeutic procedures that are often far less invasive or noninvasive. Once these technologies are adopted, they are sometimes less expensive and can be made widely available, providing access for a greater number of patients and new revenue opportunities for ambulatory physicians. Pharmaceutical advances are myriad, and genetic research is promising.

As a consequence of technology, demand-chain members are increasingly faced with the challenge of adapting to change. Long ago, general surgeons had to shift away from ulcer surgery as a major bread-and-butter service. Cardiovascular surgeons have seen a portion of their business shift to cardiologists who provide less-invasive procedures. Hospitals are seeing their inpatient, outpatient, and diagnostic business pulled away by entrepreneurial physicians backed by investment capital or their own capital. These changes place tremendous pressure on the demand chain, whose members now include providers, customers, and competitors! Managing the change process and adapting to these inevitable shifts has become an increasingly significant part of the hospital CEO's role. Maintaining relationships, balancing conflicting incentives, adapting to defections, facilitating communication, and encouraging cooperation are full-time challenges. The effort is significant and matched only by the potential benefits.

National, State, and Local Political Trends

National, state, and even some local political trends influence individual demand chains in ways similar to industries outside the healthcare arena. Local zoning ordinances; state certificate-of-need activities; state and national tort reform; the uninsured, state Medicaid programs; and many other national, state, and local issues dramatically affect the environment in which industry and healthcare organizations operate.

Take the debate over physician-owned limited-services providers such as specialty hospitals and ambulatory surgery centers. This topic has been hotly contested at the national level, and Congress has attempted to balance varying arguments from physicians and executives on both sides of the dispute. Proponents argue the benefits of increased quality and access coupled with decreased cost. Opponents argue physician conflict of interest, "cherry picking" of patients, and threats to the community healthcare safety net. Several states, with their varying levels of certificate-of-need regulation, are hearing the same arguments as they attempt to balance community need with a free-market economy. Even local governments, especially in small communities with fewer alternatives, can become embroiled in this divisive fray. As always, partisanship plays a role, as do powerful constituent and personal agendas.

Sociocultural Trends

Sociocultural trends have a significant impact on retail strategy and the demand chain. Changes in the patient/customer population and the resultant community trends now require more scrutiny than ever before. Even new physicians coming from residency programs are different from their predecessors. A significant and increasing percentage of young physicians are women wanting to balance work and family. Their male counterparts are equally driven to have a life outside of medicine. More mature physicians often complain of the different work ethic espoused by their younger partners, who also have equal or greater compensation demands. Employment has overtaken entrepreneurship as the preferred way to start practice for many graduating residents who are not keen on incurring additional debt or risk given their huge medical education loans. Offering part-time and job-share practices in addition to full-time positions is increasingly critical in competitive physician recruitment. (The financial and marketing challenges of part-time positions, in particular, are significant regardless of who owns the practice.)

The Economy

Finally, national, state, and local economies affect demand chains in every community across the nation. The rate of unemployment affects the numbers of uninsured and underinsured. National and state tax bases dramatically influence government budgets, including Medicare and Medicaid reimbursement. Healthcare expenditures continue to consume an increasing percentage of employer budgets, affecting local economies and national competitiveness. A national economic downturn has a delayed but dramatic effect on the healthcare delivery mechanism as well as on the patients we serve and the payers who pick up a portion of the tab. Even local economic bumps can have a dramatic effect on employers, employees, payers, and patients as well as on local providers of care, particularly primary care.

How primary and secondary influences will change over time and how change will affect healthcare providers are difficult to predict. However, healthcare organizations that capture market share in affiliated primary care practices and attract that market share into their demand chains will be in the best position to respond rather than react or succumb to these powerful influences.

REFERENCES

Covey, S. R. 1989. *Seven Habits of Highly Effective People: Powerful Lessons in Personal Change.* New York: Simon & Schuster.

DeNavas-Walt, C., B. D. Proctor, and C. H. Lee. 2005. *Income, Poverty, and Health Insurance Coverage in the United States: 2004.* U.S. Census Bureau, Current Population Reports, P60-229. Washington, DC: U.S. Government Printing Office.

CHAPTER 10

Creating a Culture of Accountability

This chapter presents two concepts:

- Accountability within organizations
- Accountability between organizations

As a management consultant, I come into contact with a variety of organizations, including hospitals, health systems, group practices, and medical practice networks, each with a unique culture. As an implementer of change, I become intimately acquainted with each organization's culture and its influence on the change-management process. Organizational change brings out the best and the worst in every culture. Although a few organizations actually promote change and foster performance improvement, most tend to create barriers to change—even when it is positive change. A fundamental indicator of an organization's ability to assimilate change is whether the organizational culture requires individual accountability for performance.

The success of a demand chain is highly influenced by two kinds of performance accountability. The first is accountability within each demand-chain member organization. For example, employees within a practice or a hospital department must be held accountable by management and physician leaders to meet the needs, wants, and priorities of the patient/customer or the referring physician. Retail readiness, which is discussed in Chapter 2, occurs at the individual practice or department level and requires each physician, manager, and support staff member to be individually accountable for performance. Without performance accountability at the practice or department level, activities and results are left to chance, and there is a potential negative effect on the practice or department and on the entire demand chain.

The second type of performance accountability must occur between the members of the demand chain. For example, physicians and hospital staff functioning within a service line must be accountable to each other for performance excellence. They must be willing to openly discuss performance shortfalls, to share best practices, and to change behavior to maintain demand-chain membership. The challenge of developing an accountability culture within and between demand-chain members is the subject of this chapter.

ACCOUNTABILITY DEFINED

Most healthcare organizations are reasonably effective at assigning responsibility (and good people tend to feel responsible to do a good job). Many organizations do a fairly good job of "authorizing" their team members to fulfill their responsibilities. We know who is doing what job and who is authorized to act on behalf of the organization. What many hospitals and medical practices do not do well, however, is the accountability part. We do not establish frequent and formal opportunities for individuals to "return and report," or if we do have some formal mechanism, we tend not to ask accountability questions like the following:

- Did you accomplish what you committed to?
- If not, why not? What barriers did you encounter?
- How soon will the work be accomplished?

Consequently, excellent performance is more a matter of luck, and marginal performance is more likely. Organizational leaders (physicians and managers) tend to get what they ask for in terms of accountability for individual performance.

We can learn something about accountability from sales managers. Effective sales managers have long understood the importance of frequent and specific accountability, even in environments where sales commissions are a driving force. The importance of accountability for outcomes is critical. One sales executive shared with me her experience with a very successful privately held company. Shortly after she was hired, she was invited to meet with the company president. After spending several minutes in delightful conversation, the company president shook her hand and clarified his expectations. He said, "If you can't sell, I don't need you!" She sold! While we all may not agree with the approach, the president did have a critical point that seems to escape some managers, physicians, and employees. If we do not deliver the expected results or outcomes, our organizations really do not need us, be they individual practices, hospital departments, or integrated demand chains.

Equally important is accountability for activity. In sales, cold telephone calls and other prospecting activities are difficult but essential. Many salespeople avoid cold-call prospecting like the plague, coming up with all kinds of reasons to delay or avoid the activity. Wise sales managers require a daily accounting of *activities* from each of their salespeople, knowing that if they are involved in the right activities they will be more likely to experience successful outcomes.

Clinical and nonclinical leaders of successful healthcare organizations must foster a culture that supports accountability. In fact, a culture of accountability within an organization undergirds its sustainable competitive advantage. Again, "accountability" is not the same thing as "responsibility." Accountability requires an accounting. It requires stewards to return and report the results of their stewardship. It requires leaders to make an accounting of their stewardship to followers and to the customers and communities served. Ultimately, a culture of accountability requires the demonstration of an appropriate level of performance by everyone involved in the organization. Those who are willing but fall short are assisted in every way to become successful; they may even be moved to roles more appropriate for their skills and abilities. Those who are unwilling and unable to perform are shown the door to protect patients, customers, employees, and the organization's reputation, which is the ultimate sustainable competitive advantage.

CONCEPT 1: ACCOUNTABILITY WITHIN ORGANIZATIONS[1]

Building a culture of accountability within a medical practice or a hospital department involves the following elements: effective sponsorship; a shared purpose; clear performance targets, time lines, measurement, and consequences; an effective implementation team; A-players; and weekly accountability.

Effective Sponsorship

In *Managing at the Speed of Change*, Daryl Conner (1992) defines "sponsorship" as the willingness to sanction or sponsor organizational change. Effective sponsors have not only the authority but also the will to establish direction and performance expectations for the organization based on correct principles.

Sponsorship is the most important element in creating an accountability culture. In a hospital setting, I use Conner's term "initiating sponsor" to describe the role of the CEO, as the board-appointed fiduciary, in sponsoring accountability for results. According to Conner (1992, 116), the initiating sponsor is a person who has "the power to break from the status quo and sanction a significant change." This person (most likely the hospital CEO) is supported by several other "sustaining sponsors" that likely include a governing board, medical staff leaders, a hospital executive team, and service-line or department managers who actually foster the culture of accountability. In a medical practice, the initiating sponsor may be a group president or a governing body.

In organizations with a culture of accountability, all sponsors are committed to making decisions based on proven principles of success. They make their decisions based on what is right rather than who is right or most persuasive. These exceptional leaders are authorized to make the required decisions, and they have the individual and collective will (some might say the integrity) to make even difficult choices without compromise. Once decisions are made, these leaders have the ability to establish policies in support of their decisions and to accept or assign responsibility for implementation, authorize the implementers, and hold them accountable to deliver the desired results. When barriers to implementation arise (and they always do), these leaders overcome the barriers rather than settling for something less than their organization's full potential.

A Shared Purpose

The most effective healthcare organizations possess a compelling sense of purpose that engages the physicians, management, and support staff not only in meeting the clinical needs of patients but also in identifying and meeting the nonclinical needs, wants, and priorities of their customers. Exceptional primary care practices understand that their prosperity depends on building and maintaining relationships with women, who make the majority of healthcare decisions for families. They also understand that their established female patients provide the major source of new patient referrals to the primary care practice, literally becoming the practice sales force. Exceptional specialty practices understand their need to identify and meet the needs, wants, and priorities of their customers, including Mrs. Smith and referring physicians. Exceptional hospitals and hospital-based specialists understand their shared purpose to meet the needs, wants, and priorities of patients, their families, and referring physicians.

Sponsors within these exceptional organizations not only set the service performance standards, but they also exemplify those standards and do not tolerate anything less from others within the organization. Organizational policies and procedures are built with service as a primary directive. Service issues are identified, objectively reviewed, and reported to the sponsoring body, which ensures that they receive proper management attention.

Clear Performance Targets, Time lines, Measurement, and Consequences

Successful organizations are not afraid to set significant performance targets. They strive to excel and do not leave excellence to chance, because they know chance is a poor business partner. They set performance targets and standards in the context of their common purpose to achieve both short-term and long-term objectives. These targets are documented, along with time lines for achieving them and a responsible party or parties. Lesser organizations stop at this point, satisfied that they have done all that is required for success, only to be disappointed later with their lack of achievement.

Exceptional organizations complete the process by establishing clear measurement mechanisms to assess whether progress is being made toward their objectives. Progress is reviewed frequently so barriers can be quickly identified and eliminated or managed with the help of the initiating sponsor or sponsoring body. Consequences of failure to perform are always present and consistently applied. This does not mean that an occasional misstep or failed implementation is automatic reason for dismissal or redeployment. It does mean, however, that physicians, managers, and staff who demonstrate a pattern of missed targets or standards do not remain with the organization for long.

An Effective Implementation Team

The best plans in the world are of little value if they are not effectively implemented. In every organization—from the smallest medical practice to the largest health system——initiating sponsors must depend on others to implement their plans. Governing bodies and senior leaders within organizations are accountable for the development of an effective implementation team.

In most situations, organizations delegate the responsibility for implementation to competent managers. Exceptional sponsors make sure that the manager (or management team) hired to direct implementation of approved plans and policies is also exceptional. They hire managers rather than caretakers. They expect their managers (even in the smallest medical practices) to contribute actively to performance improvement and to the implementation of best operating practices. These leaders authorize their managers to act on approved plans and direction, never undermining those managers by failing to publicly sponsor unpopular policies or procedure changes. They do not skimp on manager salaries. They know that if they hire, retain, and properly sponsor the best managers, the return on their investment will be many times the manager's compensation.

Without exception, the best-performing health systems, hospitals, and medical practices hold their managers accountable for effective implementation. They do so through frequent meetings to review performance targets, time lines, and barriers to implementation and positive outcomes.

A-Players Only Need Apply

In his book *Topgrading*, Bradford Smart (1999) discusses the significant direct and indirect costs of employing C-players. The costs include the direct financial implications of mistakes and rework, increased customer frustration and turnover, and the costs of losing frustrated A-players who have grown weary of covering for their incompetent peers. Many organizations are far too lax in their efforts to hire A-players for each position and even more hesitant to properly document poor performance and to terminate the C-players they mistakenly hire.

Exceptional organizations, on the other hand, expect their exceptional managers to hire, train, and retain the very best support staff members for each position. As Smart suggests, A-managers are not afraid to hire other A-players and are not threatened by excellent performance and innovation in their subordinates. Exceptional organizations tend to "hire slow" to identify and better match candidates with jobs. They also tend to "fire fast" when an obvious mistake has been made. These organizations make good use of a 90-day probationary period, during which they provide proper training and assess the competence of every new employee.

Weekly Accountability

Most healthcare organizations do a good job of delegating job responsibilities and authorizing employees to fulfill those responsibilities. When it comes to holding people accountable to deliver the targeted result within the approved time line, however, even sophisticated hospitals and health systems often fall short.

My colleagues and I frequently ask department and office managers a few questions related to accountability. First, we ask who holds them accountable. Most managers identify their boss. We then ask what results they are expected to achieve. This question is a bit more difficult for many. In response, we usually get a list of their job duties. When pushed a bit further regarding accountability for results, many managers either cannot respond at all or discuss their responsibility to explain budget variances (what we call "storytelling"). Finally, when we ask how they are held accountable, their responses usually reference informal discussions with the boss or a monthly meeting with organizational leaders that largely consists of coming up with a better story than the one they presented the previous month.

Accountability in exceptional organizations is different. It certainly includes a report of financial and statistical outcomes, which are often driven by the availability of information on a monthly basis. However, reporting goes well beyond quantitative outcomes to measures of qualitative performance and appropriate activity. Rather than looking in a rearview mirror 12 times each year (often three or four weeks into yet another month), effective organizations hold their valuable human resources accountable for activities much more frequently. Some activities, such as the sales force discussed earlier, lend themselves to daily accountability. In many cases, a weekly accounting of activity, progress, and barriers is adequate to ensure continued progress.

Regardless of the time frame, "if not," "why not?" and "by when?" are questions raised by sponsors in quarterly board meetings, monthly committee meetings, and senior leadership councils. They are also posed by managers to staff on a daily or weekly basis. Why weekly or more often? The answer is simple. Most of us are so busy reacting to urgent and immediate needs and demands that we fail to accomplish some of our more important tasks unless we know that we will be asked specifically about those tasks at day's end or week's end—that is, unless we will be held accountable for our activity and our outcomes.

CONCEPT 2: ACCOUNTABILITY BETWEEN ORGANIZATIONS

As if developing accountability within organizations were not difficult enough, we must also establish accountability between organizations for retail strategy and demand-chain management to work as competitive approaches. Fortunately, several principles and behaviors that foster accountability within organizations also contribute to accountability between organizations. These principles are discussed in the sections that follow.

Effective Sponsorship

Once again, the most important factor in the success or failure of a demand chain is sponsorship. Administrative and clinical leaders with the will to sponsor a shared purpose, the development of tactics based on correct principles, and accountability for demand-chain members are three factors essential to demand-chain sponsorship. Indeed, interorganizational sponsorship requires leaders with extraordinary integrity and courage. It also requires the ability to have the "crucial conversations" discussed in earlier chapters. There is no substitute for direct and respectful deliberation, debate, and communication, even regarding the toughest issues. The result of this direct and respectful communication must be a shared purpose (what the demand-chain partners will achieve) and shared tactics (how the shared purpose will be achieved) based on proven principles. The purpose and tactics must be compelling enough to attract, unite, and retain demand-chain leaders and members, especially in the face of competitive casualties and defections.

The hospital is in a unique position to serve as the integrator of demand-chain members. The success or failure of the hospital in this critical role largely depends on the CEO and her ability and credibility to serve as an initiating sponsor in the development and management of the demand chain.

A Shared Purpose

Most hospitals and health systems have a formal mission or vision statement that is supported by their sponsoring bodies, boards, senior executives, and others throughout the organization. While some physician organizations have a similar formalized statement, the mission and vision of many medical practices remain in the minds and hearts of dedicated physicians rather than being formally expressed. Although potentially powerful, common organizational mission statements are not likely to yield the type of compelling purpose needed to attract and unite demand-chain members.

A shared purpose that is compelling enough to rally the troops often involves a burning platform—even our very survival. Physicians, particularly in smaller practices, have only limited time to devote to activities that do not support next week's payroll. For example, an oncology service line consisting of physicians, administration, and support staff in multiple locations might be welded together to do battle with a large, national integrated cancer center entering the market. The stakeholders have a common and compelling purpose in combating this new competitor by working closely together to offer equivalent or better service to patients and referring physicians. Their livelihood is at stake. Physicians are more likely to join with their peers, the hospital, and others if they are doing it to ensure their continued success in the marketplace.

Clear Performance Targets, Time Lines, and Measurement

Once a shared purpose has been identified, the difficult job of developing shared demand-chain tactics must be addressed. The process of discussing and developing tactics will often solidify the demand-chain membership. Those who are not willing or not able to successfully implement the shared tactics are dropped. If their skill set is essential and no alternatives are available, the demand chain may choose to contract—at arm's length—with them to provide the service. Once tactics have been identified, performance targets or standards are established, time lines are set, and measurement mechanisms are put in place to ensure frequent peer reporting and comparison with standards.

Shared Demand-Chain Governance

While the demand chain depends on the ability of the hospital CEO as an initiating sponsor, demand-chain governance by all members is essential to the development and successful implementation of shared tactics. Whether formal or informal, the governing body must effectively sponsor the implementation of demand-chain tactics for those who choose to take part. The initiating sponsor can promote correct principles and accountability, but he cannot stand alone in promoting the success of the demand-chain. Physician members must also be involved (or see their trusted clinical peers involved) in planning, in establishing performance targets, in developing tactics, and particularly in supporting accountability throughout the demand chain.

Accountability and Consequences

The most difficult challenge in demand-chain management is holding members accountable for achieving performance targets and time lines. Accountability requires that performance data be shared openly and frequently among members. Demand-chain members should view such openness as an opportunity to help every willing member become successful by identifying performance problems and sharing best practices to improve performance. The consequences of failure must be clearly established in advance and consistently applied by a united governing body.

The most obvious potential consequence of failure by any member of the demand chain is loss of membership and the resulting referral benefits. Any corrective action involving a member of the demand chain must be fair and must be perceived as fair. Fairness usually results from the shared purpose, common tactics, clear performance targets, and consistent and accurate performance measurement. Performance improvement efforts (corrective actions) must also be clearly understood by all stakeholders. Facts are the only antidote to any perception of unfairness and should be made widely available to all demand-chain members before consequences are implemented.

Let's face it: developing a cohesive demand chain focused on a compelling purpose with members who hold each other to high standards of performance is an amazing feat. It is also an amazingly sustainable competitive advantage. This advantage has been achieved by successful heart teams, integrated oncology programs, rehabilitation service lines, and others. Such efforts often start small, with a few dedicated clinical and administrative leaders, who build on their success by adding like-minded and equally committed physicians and others until they dominate their markets.

Successful demand chains never occur by chance. They are always appropriately sponsored, always carefully managed, and always held accountable for achieving their shared purpose through shared tactics. Successful demand-chain members share a culture of commitment and a willingness to *be* accountable, without which there is no chance for success. Are successful demand chains difficult to achieve? Yes. Are they sustainable as a competitive advantage? Absolutely!

NOTE

1. This concept originally appeared in Marc D. Halley. 2005. " A Culture of Accountability: What Distinguishes an Exceptional Medical Group." *Group Practice Journal* 54 (3): 10–14. Reprinted with permission from the *Group Practice Journal*. Copyright © 2005, American Medical Group Association.

REFERENCES

Conner, D. R. 1992. *Managing at the Speed of Change: How Resilient Managers Succeed and Prosper Where Others Fail.* New York: Villard Books.

Smart, B. D. 1999. *Topgrading: How Leading Companies Win by Hiring, Coaching and Keeping the Best People.* New York: Prentice Hall Press.

CHAPTER 11

A Sustainable Competitive Advantage

This chapter presents six concepts:

- Trust
- The right plan
- Long-term commitment
- Degree of difficulty
- Relationships
- A culture of accountability

Winning in the competitive healthcare arena gets more difficult every year. Hospitals and physicians continue to adapt to industry changes and challenges, but few avoid some level of pain and suffering. In certain markets, profits still support capital accumulation and competitive physician incomes. Elsewhere, physicians and hospitals struggle to stay even, and sheer will and commitment to their communities drive them to hang on.

In the midst of industry regulations, increasing competition, decreasing reimbursement, malpractice crises, limited-services providers, and other concerns, remembering our fundamental purpose is difficult: to create and keep a customer.

Regardless of the market situation, short-term and long-term success require that demand chains capture and retain not only the allegiance of the retail customer but also a cadre of PCPs and the right specialists to meet community health needs and support distinct service lines. When we achieve equality with competing demand chains, we earn a temporary seat at the competitive table. But doing a better job guarantees market-share growth and a long-term position in our communities. Likewise, failure to at least match competing demand chains ensures a slow but steady decline for the hospital and its affiliated medical staff members.

My physician practice management company works with some clients who have achieved competitive advantage and now lead their markets. We also work with others who are second or third in the competitive game. As an integral part of our work, we interview CEOs and other senior executives regarding their competitors' strengths and weaknesses. We have found that characterizing our more powerful competitors as villains who have tremendous unearned advantages is human nature. A huge "war chest," a better location, a more cooperative medical staff, local political advantage, and other factors are viewed by senior executives on the other side of the fence as "free gifts," as if to discount the competitor's success.

In the long run every demand chain has a similar set of potential competitive strategies and tactics. Even those who are trailing in market share can outmaneuver better-positioned rivals over time. It all comes down to the right targets, the right process, and the right execution. We consistently find that the key to success is implementing the right tactics day by day, week by week, and year by year, and this is the topic of this final chapter.

When is a competitive advantage truly sustainable? If all demand chains potentially have the same strategies and tactics over the long run, how can any single competitor sustain an advantage over others in the marketplace? We propose that sustainability derives from several key factors:

- Trust
- The right plan
- Long-term commitment
- Degree of difficulty
- Relationships
- A culture of accountability

CONCEPT 1: TRUST

Few things are worse in the workplace than not being able to trust one's boss. It is difficult at best to follow the lead of one whose motivations, actions, or words are inconsistent and questionable. Too many executives, both experienced and inexperienced, avoid the straight talk that is needed in a good partnership with physicians (or anyone else for that matter). I have seen executives struggle to come up with the right spin on tough messages because they "don't want to make the doctors mad." This tactic may avoid a negative response in the short run, but doctors are highly intelligent people. They will know when they have been had. Then the executive will still be faced with the same harsh reality but with no credibility to communicate it or to engage physicians in finding and implementing a solution. Trust me—the positive spin tactic never works for long!

Trustworthiness is more than just telling the truth. It involves introspection and the ability to admit mistakes or our own contribution to poor decisions. It also involves vulnerability—a willingness to patiently endure those who continually bully their way around medical staff or department meetings, operating rooms, or hospital hallways. It involves taking occasional hits but not flinching from one's commitment to principles. Trustworthiness requires a commitment to the organization, to physicians, and to partners and a genuine concern about the people affected by decisions, particularly negative ones. Finally, trustworthiness requires "putting one's capital where one's mouth is." It means having the integrity to stay the course when faced with challenges to the shared vision.

CONCEPT 2: THE RIGHT PLAN

The right plan is based on correct principles. It creates and helps keep customers, rallies the troops, and presents a clear end game. To develop the right plan, we must be willing to understand the organization's current circumstances. We must be rigorous in assessing the organization's strengths and weaknesses in terms of current and anticipated competitive offerings. At hospital and demand-chain planning sessions, my colleagues and I frequently see comments such as "We have the best doctors in town" listed among organizations' strengths. When pressed, however, few organizations can prove the validity of such a statement. A legitimate planning process does not accept such unsubstantiated perceptions, because they may mask a weakness or exclude a potential market opportunity.

Plan development also requires an in-depth understanding of the retail market and apparent competitor strategies. With accurate information about environmental trends (e.g., technology, the economy, legal/regulatory issues, and demographic data), opportunities and threats can be identified, leading to a valid discussion of the end game and the development of a legitimate vision. By "legitimate vision" I mean one that is relevant to capturing and retaining market share, as opposed to a vision statement, which too often is grounded in platitudes. Writing a "possible organization paper" (POP) is a good way to capture that vision by clearly defining the target market and documenting a specific strategy for capturing that market. (Appendix C shows a sample POP.) The POP outlines which strategies and tactics will be implemented, based on a clear picture of the organization and the rules for success in that business. Once the vision is clear, we can develop strategies (objectives/directions) and tactics (methods) to achieve the POP.

A vision of the organization that has the power to capture the hearts and minds of our physician partners cannot be solely about the hospital. It must be about the demand chain, and there must be clear potential for all involved to win. Such a vision requires the hands and hearts of those who will champion the development of the demand chain. Of course, we might be concerned that engaging physicians, management, and staff in this process will heighten the risk that our competitors will know our strategies sooner than we do. In reality, however, the success of a legitimate vision depends not on secrecy but on skilled execution. Our vision will become apparent through our strategies and tactics, so it will soon be on the radar of any interested and aggressive competitor. Because successful implementation of the vision requires ownership by all key stakeholders—physicians and staff alike—engaging them throughout the developmental process is vital. It is worth the risk.

CONCEPT 3: LONG-TERM COMMITMENT

The gap between our vision, as represented in a POP, and our current reality will not be bridged by any single event. Even the greatest speech by a gifted CEO will do little more than raise interest among some and anxiety in others. We will only bridge the gap by identifying a clear pathway and process for all persons affected by the strategies and tactics. The most significant and sustainable competitive vision, strategies, and tactics take tremendous effort and, most importantly, time. In a world in which so many executives worship at the altar of monthly or quarterly financial results, the CEO (or initiating sponsor) must be tremendously committed to be able to stay the course.

Physicians often complain to me about the short tenure of many hospital executives and the resulting changes in course, pace, and focus as each new CEO or service-line leader implements her priorities. Turnover is indeed costly in terms of competitive advantage. New leaders are often hailed as saviors, as if to justify the organization's hiring decision. Some organizations expect big change when a new CEO comes to town, and new leaders may find themselves too anxious to place their mark on the organization—to the detriment of critical strategic momentum.

The winners in the competitive battle operate differently. Sustaining sponsors (Conner 1992)—such as board members, system executives, medical staff leaders, and the hospital management team—protect a carefully selected vision, strategies, and tactics. They are loathe to change. Course corrections certainly occur, but they are driven by changes in the marketplace or actual implementation experience and performance feedback. The result is a long-term commitment to vision and direction, even though a few zig-zags may appear in the implementation process. By contrast, market losers constantly make 90-degree and 180-degree course corrections based on the whim of rotating leadership.

CONCEPT 4: DEGREE OF DIFFICULTY

I am always intrigued by the precise twists and turns of competitive divers, whether in the near-perfect arena of the Olympics or the less consistent platform of college and high school diving teams. The judges' scores represent both the diver's execution and the degree of difficulty of the selected dive. The champion divers execute the toughest dives with near-perfect consistency. In some respects, achieving a sustainable competitive advantage in healthcare requires the same consistent execution and a high degree of difficulty to ward off less courageous competitors.

A sustainable competitive advantage is always difficult to achieve. Therefore, replicating it is difficult because it involves significant work and risk. Very often, risky strategies are associated with capital expenditures. Bricks-and-mortar projects represent long-term commitments. When organizations have huge treasure chests, long-term strategies may be enough, especially where certificate-of-need regulation protects service lines. But in the long term, capital-based strategies actually are quite vulnerable. A competitor with money (readily available from a number of sources) can enter a market or strike from within to steal away profitable services or entire service lines. This pilfering can occur even in certificate-of-need states.

CONCEPT 5: RELATIONSHIPS

The most competitive strategies are based on relationships with and among talented people. Regardless of available capital, the clinical quality, customer service, and product innovations provided by a talented team of people are difficult to match. Members of such teams are not necessarily on the same payroll, but they have developed a common vision and commitment to excellence. Successful teams may occur at the board level, among senior management, within the medical staff, in the operating room, or at the department level. Wherever they are found, they share these characteristics:

- *Intelligence.* Intelligent people who work together are definitely vital to sustainable competitive advantage. Intelligent professionals must be sought out and retained. Successful competitors rigorously pursue A-players, who represent the finest talent available for the dollars the organization is able to pay (Smart 1999). Equally important is the difficult challenge of removing C-players, who sap the life out of departments and organizations. Difficult? Yes. Worth it? Yes!
- *Skills and talent.* Raw intelligence must be combined with natural talent and acquired skills to ensure that clinical and other services provided to both internal and external customers are of unequalled quality. Hiring and retaining a talented team takes much more than money. An engaging vision, great leadership, and the freedom to pursue one's potential are also critical.
- *Mutual respect.* There is no room and precious little tolerance for prima donnas on successful teams. Yes, team members

should have the utmost respect for physicians, who have trained many years to develop their knowledge and skills. At the same time, those talented physicians must give mutual respect to the support teams, without whom they could not apply their talents as effectively and efficiently as they do. A culture built on mutual respect must start at the top and will not put up with anything less throughout the rank and file of the organization.

- *Dialog.* In *Crucial Conversations*, Patterson and colleagues (2002) discuss the critical contribution of communication to the success of organizations and the quality of their services. The authors also discuss the dangers posed by failing to communicate with patients. The ability to discuss tough issues, openly and respectfully in a safe environment, is essential to patient care in the short term and to a sustainable competitive advantage in the long run. Developing the ability to hold "crucial conversations" is difficult, but the return on the effort and risk can be phenomenal.

- *Introspection/learning.* In *The Fifth Discipline*, Peter Senge (1999) emphasizes the essential skill of organizational learning. The ability to learn and adapt as individuals, teams, departments, and organizations has never been more important than it is in today's highly competitive healthcare environment. The willingness of teams to be introspective, supported by the ability to engage in dialog, results in the objective review of outcomes and true performance improvement—and sometimes even in breakthrough innovation. Easy to achieve? Not a chance! But essential nonetheless.

- *Quality focus.* To attract and retain customers while warding off competitors, the organization's focus, both internally and externally, must be on high-quality clinical care and high-quality customer service. No amount of advertising can overcome less-than-stellar performance. As individuals, teams, departments, and organizations, we must not merely discuss and measure but actually and consistently produce high-quality outcomes. Only then can we attain a sustainable competitive advantage.

The bottom line is only people and teams can create a competitive advantage that is likely to be sustainable in the marketplace.

CONCEPT 6: A CULTURE OF ACCOUNTABILITY

Leaders of successful organizations foster a culture of accountability, which requires years of consistent leadership and effort. Developing a culture of accountability is the foundation for achieving a sustainable competitive advantage.

Do not confuse "accountability" with the feeling of "responsibility" held by most good people. Accountability requires an accounting. It requires stewards to return and report the results of their stewardship at every level within the organization. It requires leaders to document their stewardship to followers and to the customers and communities served. Ultimately, a culture of accountability requires the demonstration of an appropriate level of performance for everyone involved in the organization. Those willing individuals who fall short are assisted in every way to improve their performance. The unwilling and unable are shown the door to protect the organization's patients, customers, employees, and reputation—and that is the ultimate sustainable competitive advantage.

REFERENCES

Conner, D. R. 1992. *Managing at the Speed of Change*. New York: Villard Books.

Patterson, K., J. Grenny, R. McMillan, A. Switzler, and S. Covey. 2002. *Crucial Conversations: Tools for Talking When Stakes Are High*. New York: McGraw-Hill.

Senge, P. M. 1990. *The Fifth Discipline: The Art & Practice of the Learning Organization*. New York: Currency Doubleday.

Smart, B. D. 1999. *Topgrading: How Leading Companies Win by Hiring, Coaching and Keeping the Best People*. New York: Prentice Hall Press.

Retail Readiness Evaluation

©2006 The Halley Consulting Group, LLC

Customer Knowledge	● Yes ○ No

1. We have sorted our customer population by zip code to better understand our draw area. ☐
2. We track how our new patients learn about our practice/provider. ☐
3. Our computer system is set up to track demographic data such as patient age, sex, marital status, family size, employment status, and address. ☐
4. Our computer system is set up to track classes of chronic clinical diagnoses such as diabetes and asthma. ☐
5. We can sort our customer database by demographic and/or clinical diagnosis categories. ☐
6. We track the reasons why our customers leave our practice. ☐
7. We routinely ask our patients how we performed on their most recent visit to our office. ☐
8. We ask our patients what additional services they would like us to offer. ☐
9. We ask our patients what information they would like about their health and medical care. ☐
10. We identify the needs, wants, and priorities of our customers and make them part of our training and process improvement efforts. ☐

11. We have a suggestion box in our reception room and in our exam rooms to solicit customer comments and concerns. ☐

12. Periodically we formally survey both active and inactive customers to supplement the knowledge gained by surveying our frequent visitors. ☐

13. We contact our patients about their satisfaction with the providers to whom we refer them for services since these referent physicians reflect on our image. ☐

14. Our physicians, management, and staff routinely discuss the results of our surveys and suggestions and develop action plans to address practice problems and to take advantage of positive suggestions. ☐

Customer Knowledge: Total capabilities identified =

(Count each ● Yes)

Customer Access ● Yes ○ No

15. We offer extended hours for the convenience of our customers. ☐

16. We offer weekend hours for the convenience of our customers. ☐

17. We are able to accommodate all requests for acute appointments every day. ☐

18. We track our ability to respond to a customer's first and second requests for an appointment. ☐

19. We answer the telephone by the third ring. ☐

20. We never leave a patient on hold more than 30 seconds. ☐

21. As an alternative to placing a customer on hold, we offer to have the appointment desk return calls within 15 minutes. ☐

22. Our appointment desk offers other practice providers as options if the requested provider is not available. ☐

23. Our appointment desk offers other network providers if our providers are unavailable. ☐

24. Our providers have a liberal "work-in" policy. ☐

25. We use wave scheduling or open access scheduling alternatives. ☐

26. We use mid-level providers to handle acute cases that our physicians cannot work into their schedules. ☐

27. Our appointment desk is trained to ask appropriate questions in order to schedule adequate time for the requested visit. ☐

28. Patients can find our office easily because we are all trained to provide clear directions from main thoroughfares throughout our community. ☐

Customer Access: Total capabilities identified =

(Count each ● Yes)

Customer Expectations	● Yes ○ No

29. We promote "get acquainted" visits to new customers at no charge. ☐

30. We have a practice brochure that explains our policies and answers frequently asked questions, including ways to reach us after hours, how to handle prescription refills, and financial matters. ☐

31. We send Welcome Packets to new customers in advance of their first visit. ☐

32. In addition to taking a patient's vital signs and noting the chief complaint, our clinical staff always asks the patient what his or her objectives are for the visit and notes those objectives for the provider. ☐

33. Our providers note the patient's objectives for the visit in their initial communication with the patient upon entering the exam room. ☐

Customer Expectations: Total capabilities identified =

(Count each ● Yes)

34. We hire outgoing, friendly staff members who view customer service as part of their personal mission in life. ☐
35. Our current staff members recommend new hires they think will "fit" our customer-focused culture. ☐
36. Each of our staff members receives formal training in customer service techniques. ☐
37. All staff members go through a formal customer service training process annually. ☐
38. Our staff members frequently receive unsolicited cards, letters, and other compliments from patients regarding their quality of care. ☐
39. Customer service is one of the critical factors in every staff member's performance appraisal. ☐
40. All of our staff members are well trained in their technical role within the practice. Trainees are identified for customers. ☐

Customer Service Team: Total capabilities identified =

(Count each ● Yes)

41. We have established a customer "bill of rights" expressing our commitment to our patients and their families. ☐
42. We place our customer "bill of rights" in various places throughout our practice in order to educate our patients and remind ourselves of our commitments. ☐
43. We openly display nice photos of our providers and staff members along with our commitment to patient caring in the reception room. A nice notebook containing photos and brief biographies of our providers and staff members is also available for customer review in our reception area. ☐
44. We hold weekly staff meetings and discuss customer service as one of the agenda items. ☐

45. We hold periodic "brown bag lunches" to process improve each step in the customer service process. ☐
46. We are always "experimenting" to improve the experience of our patients and customers. ☐
47. Staff members are encouraged to look for examples of caring customer service provided by their peers. ☐
48. We have a set of "rewards" to celebrate examples of outstanding customer service on the part of staff and physicians. ☐
49. Our physicians routinely compliment staff members for their customer service orientation. ☐
50. We occasionally use a "mystery shopper" to test our performance. The mystery shopper completes a formal survey, which is provided to the office manager for discussion during a staff meeting. ☐
51. We track customer flow through the practice tenaciously! We understand and overcome bottlenecks that cause our customers to wait for service. ☐
52. Our providers use "social progress" notes in the chart to help them remember special thoughts, children and grandchildren, hobbies, vacations, special events, accomplishments, and concerns shared by customers in the exam room. The provider and staff in Welcome Letters, when refilling prescriptions, and on subsequent visits reference these social notes or non-medical history. ☐

Customer Service Culture: Total capabilities identified =

(Count each ● Yes)

Customer Service Policies	● Yes ○ No

53. Managers and providers compliment in public and provide negative feedback in private. ☐
54. Yes, in our practice the customer is still always right. ☐
55. We never cancel a customer's appointment with us—ever! ☐
56. We never talk about patients or customers in negative terms. ☐
57. The first staff member to hear a customer's concern owns that concern until it is resolved. ☐

58. Owners complete an incident card on every complaint for review during staff meetings. ☐

59. We use patient and customer names in addressing them, whenever possible. ☐

60. Every patient deserves a smile, whether in person or on the telephone. ☐

61. In order to ensure customer comfort, serving as a chaperone is a clinical assistant's top priority, even if exam rooms are left open for brief periods of time. ☐

62. We staff our office to keep receptionists "receiving" and clinical assistants "assisting," thereby maximizing the customer's experience and the provider's productivity. ☐

63. Every customer complaint receives a signed letter from the provider apologizing for the frustration, discussing how the issue is being corrected, and asking the customer to provide additional feedback on the next visit. This letter is kept in front of the customer's chart so the clinical assistant and the provider can solicit comments during the next visit. ☐

64. Our network monitors common drug and supply costs at various pharmacies in our market area to share with our customers in order to save them money. They publish this information for our offices. ☐

Customer Service Policies: Total capabilities identified =

(Count each ● Yes)

Education/Promotion ● Yes ○ No

65. Our computer system can create mailing lists for our customer population or subsets of that population. ☐

66. We have developed or acquired patient education information on topics of importance to our customers, which we distribute upon request in the exam room. ☐

67. We stratify our customer population based upon age and sex in order to provide education materials and encourage appropriate physical and screening examinations. ☐

68. We have a designated receptionist who follows up on screening campaigns to set up appointments for interested customers. ☐

69. Our customers know that we are interested in their referrals of friends and relatives. ☐

70 We have implemented a referral reward system for customers who refer their friends and relatives to us. ☐

71. We use "personalized" Welcome Letters for every new patient, including the doctor's signature and personal comment. ☐

72. Our providers are active in promoting health education in the local community through speaking engagements, articles written for lay publications, radio and television interviews, health fairs, and other occasions. Part of our office manager's responsibility is to facilitate these opportunities. ☐

73. Our clinical assistants give educational materials to customers in the exam room based upon their requests. Our providers note customers' interests and provide additional educational materials based upon their diagnosis(es). These educational materials are made available through our network and professional affiliations. ☐

74. Each day our providers identify and spend 15 minutes calling certain "key" patients, personally. Those key patients may include family members, other professionals, those expressing particular concerns about a diagnosis or referral, etc. ☐

75. We routinely use statement stuffers as an avenue to provide education and personal messages for our customers. ☐

76. Our providers and staff members recognize the potential for customer referral in every human interaction, including pharmacists, hospital administration and staff, insurers, drug reps, and others. All are treated with dignity and respect. ☐

77. We have a well-designed advertisement in the Yellow Pages. ☐

78. We direct mail or participate with Welcome Wagon or other agencies that greet new patients moving to our market. ☐

Education/Promotion: Total capabilities identified =

(Count each ● Yes)

Customer Experience   ● Yes ○ No

79. Every customer is greeted by a warm smile within seconds of entering our office. ☐

80. We do not separate our receptionist from our customers by glass or any other barrier. ☐
81. We provide soft music in our reception room. ☐
82. Our reception room is always clean and comfortable. ☐
83. We provide a telephone in our reception area for patients to use in making local calls. ☐
84. We set **short** "wait" time objectives, report our average "wait" time to our customers, and commit to reducing that wait time. ☐
85. We "manage" our reception room by communicating with our customers frequently, particularly if the provider is running behind. Our customers never need to guess. ☐
86. Our receptionist completes a short reception room evaluation at least once each day. ☐
87. We provide a variety of current reading materials for our adult customers and frequently cleaned toys for our young patients. ☐
88. Our examination rooms are always clean and comfortable. ☐
89. Our clinical assistants "manage" their assigned exam rooms by communicating frequently with customers awaiting the provider. Communication includes their position in the line. ☐
90. When a customer must disrobe for the examination we always offer a cloth gown. ☐
91. We provide a private area for our customers to discuss financial matters and schedule follow-up appointments with our cashier. ☐
92. We warmly thank each of our customers for coming to see us "today." ☐
93. We recognize the accounts receivable management process as part of the customer's experience with our office. Our entire process, including pre-collections, maintains the dignity of the customer. ☐

Customer Experience: Total capabilities identified =

(Count each ● Yes)

Retail Practice Evaluation Scores (Transfer totals from previous sections)	
Customer Knowledge	
Customer Access	
Customer Expectations	
Customer Service Team	
Customer Service Culture	
Customer Service Policies	
Education/Promotion	
Customer Experience	
Total	
Overall Score ÷ 93 x 100 = (Rounded to the nearest whole number)	

Pro Forma for a Cold-Start Practice

Following is an example of a pro forma that illustrates how a cold-start practice might grow during a two-year time frame.

Year 1 Pro Forma		Month 1	Month 2	Month 3	....	Total Yr 1
Volume and Revenue						
Patient volume/day		5	5	6	....	
Patient volume/mo (based on 4.5 days/wk, 4 wk/mo)		90	90	108	....	
Gross charges (based on $110 per patient)		9,900	9,900	11,880	....	211,860
Total net revenue (based on 70% collection ratio)		6,930	6,930	8,316	....	148,302
Nonphysician Expenses						
Variable expenses (med. supplies, etc.)		1,386	1,386	1,663	....	29,660
Nonphys. wages and benefits		9,804	9,804	9,804	....	117,650
Subtotal fixed expense (rent, ins., equip., etc.)		5,046	5,046	5,046	....	60,550
Net Income Before Physician(s)		498	498	1,607	....	58,092
Physician Expenses						
	Annual Values					
Physician compensation	140,000.00	11,667	11,667	11,667	....	140,000
Physician benefits (20% of compensation)	28,000.00	2,053	2,053	2,053	....	24,634
Total compensation and benefits	168,000.00	13,719	13,719	13,719	....	164,634
Net Income (loss) After Physician Comp. and Benefits		(26,941)	(26,941)	(25,832)	....	**(271,176)**

....	Month 22	Month 23	Month 24	Total Yr 2
....	26	27	28	
....	468	486	504	
....	51,480	53,460	55,440	512,820
....	36,036	37,422	38,808	358,974
....	7,207	7,484	7,762	71,795
....	9,804	9,804	9,804	117,650
....	5,183	5,183	5,183	62,200
....	23,645	24,754	25,863	224,979
....	11,667	11,667	11,667	140,000
....	2,053	2,053	2,053	24,634
....	13,719	13,719	13,719	164,634
....	(3,794)	(2,685)	(1,576)	(104,288)

Example of a Possible Organization Paper (POP)

Horton Hospital owns and operates a physician network, serving patients in key locations throughout Watson County. We have an employed or affiliated primary care physician or mid-level provider within a ten-minute drive of most neighborhoods within our primary market and within a 20-minute drive for many families in our secondary market. Our network's geographic coverage has made us indispensable to payers contracting with patients and employers in our market area. Payers recognize our "brand" and the fact that we must be included in any viable insurance plan offering in our market. Consequently, we have more than adequate access to patients for our primary care retail outlets.

Our physician network is part of a unique partnership between hospital leadership and employed physicians. We have built that partnership on the basis of mutual trust. That trust has developed as we have made decisions together. We understand that our partnership must ensure the viability of the primary care physicians, our affiliated specialists, and the hospital, if we are to prosper. We work together in a timely way to identify decision alternatives, to understand the implications of those alternatives, and to make the best decision possible to strengthen our demand chain over the long run. On those few occasions when it becomes clear that we have made a poor decision, we trust each other enough to jointly own and solve the problem. As a result of our relationship, we have become the premier physician/hospital partnership in the region. Other partnerships around the country are basing their partnership development on our approach.

We have worked with our staff to develop a high level of clinical quality and service quality, which distinguishes us from our competitors. Our culture promotes excellent medical care, delivered effectively and efficiently. Our culture also ensures that we deliver that medical care in a caring manner, as defined and recognized by our patients. We measure our performance in both of these critical areas, and we publish the results to our current and potential patients, employers, and insurance carriers. Our clinical and service quality promote our "brand" within the community and ensure that our physicians experience high patient-referral volume, which can build current or new practices.

We offer a wide array of services in our primary care sites, based on the needs, wants, and priorities of our patient population. We track those patient needs, wants, and priorities and develop innovative products and services to make our practice sites more convenient, attractive, and accessible than those of our competition. While not extravagant, our sites are pleasantly appointed and well equipped.

Physicians, hospital leadership, and staff all recognize the importance of financial viability in continuing to offer our high-quality "care and caring" to the community. We have worked together to ensure that each of our practice sites operates at the financial break-even point, or better. The only exceptions to this standard are sites where we are making a strategic investment or sites where mission objectives make financial performance a secondary priority. However, even in these sites we are wise stewards of our financial resources.

We recognize that people are our most important asset. We place great emphasis on hiring people who want to grow with us, we train them well and continuously, we give them opportunities to advance, and we pay them fairly for their efforts. We offer a wage and benefits package that is competitive with other medical practice offerings in our community. Our training and advancement opportunities, however, set us apart from the competition.

We have a strong management team at the network and practice-site levels. Each individual is a well-trained and capable implementer of decisions made by the partnership. Continuous training and communication ensures that best practices are quickly isolated and shared among our network sites, as approved by our physician and nonphysician leadership. A full-time controller and a full-time central processing manager support our management team.

We have invested in the infrastructure necessary to support effective and efficient decision making at the strategic and operating levels. Our billing system is current and fully capable and is integrated with our electronic medical record. Our financial and statistical reporting is accurate and timely.

Our physician network has become a sustainable competitive advantage to the hospital and a tremendous benefit to the medical staff in general. In addition to helping the hospital more effectively meet its mission, the network has directly increased our share of the market and made us clearly the dominant competitor.

About the Author

Marc D. Halley, M.B.A., has been working with hospitals and medical practices since 1984. He was a founding partner and the managing partner of Lexus Management Corporation, which provided interim management and consulting services to medical practices/networks and medical staff development planning for hospitals until 1991. Mr. Halley joined Holy Cross Health Services of Utah in 1991 and served in hospital and system roles. In 1995 he worked with Holy Cross Health System Corporation to start Ambulatory Management Services, Inc. (AMS), which specialized in working with hospital-owned medical practices and primary care practice networks. After the merger of Holy Cross Health System Corporation and Mercy Health Services in 2000, AMS became part of the resulting Trinity Health.

In 2005 Mr. Halley formed The Halley Consulting Group, LLC. Halley Consulting is the result of Mr. Halley's many years of providing medical staff development, practice management, and consulting services to hospital-owned and private medical practices.

Mr. Halley is a frequently requested speaker and lecturer, addressing national conferences, governing boards, senior executives, physician groups, and management teams. He has authored and coauthored several articles published in healthcare industry magazines and journals. Mr. Halley received a B.S. in business administration–management from Weber State College (now University) and an M.B.A. from Utah State University. He and his wife, Debbie, are the parents of six children and a golden retriever.